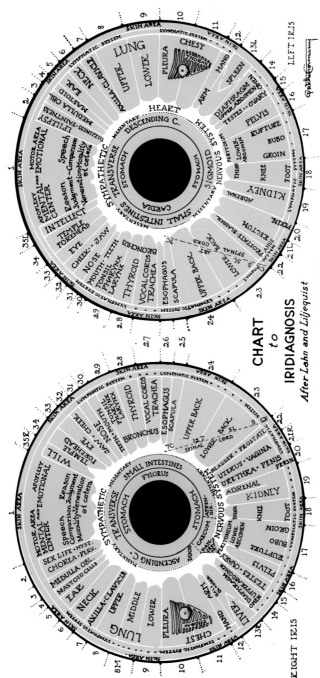

CHART
to
IRIDIAGNOSIS

After Lahn and Liljequist

Revised by Henry Lindlahr, M.D.

NATURAL THERAPEUTICS
VOLUME FOUR

IRIDIAGNOSIS
AND OTHER
DIAGNOSTIC METHODS

HENRY LINDLAHR, MD
Edited and Revised by

JOCELYN C.P. PROBY
M.A., M.Litt (Oxon), D.O. (Kirksville, U.S.A.)

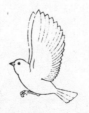

SAFFRON WALDEN
THE C.W. DANIEL COMPANY LTD

First published in this edition by
The C.W. Daniel Company Limited
1 Church Path, Saffron Walden, Essex, CB10 1JP, England

ISBN 85207 171 X

©Henry Lindlahr 1919
Revisions and Additions ©Jocelyn C.P. Proby 1985

Printed in Great Britain by
Hillman Printers (Frome) Ltd, Frome, Somerset

ACKNOWLEDGEMENTS

The editor wishes to acknowledge the extensive help given by Farida Davidson, director of the new British School of Natural Medicine and director too of the British School of Iridology, Bright Haven, Robin's Lane, Lolworth, Cambridge, England.

CONTENTS

EDITOR'S INTRODUCTION

When published in Dr. Lindlahr's lifetime this volume on the subject of Iridiagnosis was numbered by him as Volume VI in the series. The reason for this was that he wished it to be looked upon as the last volume of the series although it was finished and put into print before Volumes IV and V which, it appears, were in preparation but were never actually published before his death. Thus we know that the series is incomplete and that we are deprived of the ideas and information which Lindlahr intended to impart in the two missing volumes and to which he refers in a number of passages in the four volumes which we do possess. All we know about the missing volumes is that he intended Volume IV to be entitled "Eugenics, or Man Building on the Physical, Mental and Moral Planes of Being" and Volume V to discuss the nature and treatment of certain special diseases of a grave and difficult character, contrasting the approach of Natural Therapeutics with that of orthodox medicine. It is perhaps in the Practice and the Iridiagnosis volumes that one is most aware of a certain incompleteness and deficiency in what is being said on certain subjects which he apparently meant to deal with more fully in the missing volumes. In these cases I have tried to insert notes and appendices which may be helpful to those studying his works.

This volume falls into several parts. In the first six chapters Lindlahr gives something of the history of Iridiagnosis, an outline of the anatomy, histology and physiology of the eye and of the iris and an explanation of the manner in which the signs in the iris are produced. In the next fifteen chapters there is detailed information on the interpretation of the signs including the abnormal colouring which is imparted to the iris by drugs and poisons taken into the body by accident or by medication of the orthodox allopathic kind. Two chapters are then devoted to a discussion of the ductless glands, their secretions, their interrelations one with another, their diseases and the methods by which those diseases should be treated. Finally, he deals with the system or technique known as "basic diagnosis" which he claims to be a very useful means of obtaining a more complete diagnostic picture in difficult chronic cases and to be particularly helpful in arriving at a sound prognosis. The book is very profusely illustrated with pictures and drawings, some of which are in colour, which makes for a much better understanding both of the technique of Iridiagnosis and of the numerous case reports which are given in the text.

Taking the work as a whole, it speaks for itself, but attention may be drawn to a number of points. First, it is impossible to read it without feeling how immensely important it is that the study and use of Iridiagnosis should not be allowed to lapse or disappear. It is clear that an intelligent study and use of this method is capable of adding a new dimension to the art and practice of diagnosis and prognosis. It is true that considerable advances in diagnostic procedures and techniques have been made since Lindlahr's time both in the orthodox medical world and by exponents of electronic and radionic methods; yet it is difficult not to feel that there is something quite unique and unrivalled in the ability which Lindlahr acquired to obtain a picture in his mind of the condition and functioning ability of a person's body and its organs at any given moment, to put his finger on the causes of the body having come into that condition and to assess the possibilities for the future. Undoubtedly Iridiagnosis has, or should have, a great part to play in diagnosis in the future though it should not, as Lindlahr himself says, be used exclusively, but in combination with other useful diagnostic methods which exist or which may be developed. It must, however, be noted that though it is highly desirable that Iridiagnosis should be accepted more widely it will be no easy task to bring this about. The reason is that the truths which Iridiagnosis reveals condemn absolutely a very large proportion of the treatment which is being given by the orthodox medical profession at the present time. What is in fact being done on a very wide scale is to suppress acute disease by the wrong sort of treatment and turn it into chronic disease to the accompaniment of a poisoning of the body by every kind of chemical which is alien to it and cannot easily be eliminated. This way of proceeding has the support of learned establishments and medical schools and is tied up with the uncritical acceptance of the germ theory of disease in a crude Pasteurian form and the development of an elaborate science or pseudo-science of pharmacology. Behind all this there is an enormous international chemical and pharmaceutical industry which is immensely rich and powerful and which has, to a great extent, become the master and not the servant of the doctors and medical scientists, though the doctors and scientists are not generally aware of the fact. It may, therefore, be predicted that it will be a difficult task to obtain sympathetic consideration or acceptance of Iridiagnosis and of the conclusions to which its use and study are bound to lead in the realms of medical thought and practice. On the other hand, it may be noted that the physiological mechanism by which Iridiagnosis appears to work has an affinity with such things as acupuncture, spondylotherapy and reflex and zonal therapies which depend on the existence in the body of nerve connections and pathways by which conditions in one part of the body can be detected or influenced by means of reflexes initiated in another part. This should perhaps cause Iridiagnosis to be more acceptable in certain quarters.

Secondly, Iridiagnosis vindicates Lindlahr's contention that chemicals in crude inorganic form should not, as a general rule, be used in the treatment of disease. These substances are in fact protoplasmic poisons and the effects which they have are not, and cannot be, curative, but are to be regarded as being in the realms of toxicology. Moreover it is shown by Iridiagnosis that they tend in different degrees to be retained in the body in parts or areas for which they have an affinity and there to produce irritation, malfunction and deterioration of tissue. Some of the case reports which Lindlahr gives are not only of outstanding interest but are quite horrifying as revealing the terrible harm which can be done unwittingly by honest and well-meaning people, and the extent to which chronic disease is being created by doctors and pharmacists. Whether this is as much so as it was in Lindlahr's time is hard to say but, though there has been real progress in some branches of medicine, it is not easy to be sure that most doctors do not create more disease than they cure. This is because so much treatment is symptomatic and not directed to the causes behind the symptoms. This is bound to be harmful in most cases because the symptoms are not the disease and do in fact often represent the effort of the body to rid itself of the disease. It is also because there seems to be a very curious sort of "double think" about drugs. When they are studied under the name of toxicology the harmful effects which they can produce are often well understood and set forth, but when they are studied under the umbrella of pharmacology or materia medica this is all largely forgotten and their supposed benefits and usefulness in various disease conditions are praised and recommended. This might not matter so much if the drugs used were harmless in themselves and were quickly and easily eliminated from the body after having performed a useful function in it, but Lindlahr makes it very clear in his case reports and in his analyses of the various drugs commonly used in medical practice, that this is not the case. It may be stated as a general rule and principle that when drugs are used with apparent success they are suppressing and not curing the disease and that they tend not to be eliminated easily or quickly even when administered in small doses, but rather to accumulate in the body, often in the most vital organs, and to produce malfunction, destruction of tissue and chronic disease, often of the most terrible kind. It must be conceded that there are a few cases and situations in which certain drugs can legitimately be used as, for instance, for anaesthesia or to relieve intolerable pain until a patient can be got to a place where a good kind of care and treatment can be initiated, but these situations need not be very common and should become less so as our skill and knowledge increases. For instance, there are signs that there are some methods of anaesthesia being developed which do not entail the administration of drugs and Lindlahr affirms that the control of pain by natural methods of treatment is nearly always more effective and happier for the patient than the continuous use of drugs and pain killers, even in such conditions as terminal cancer.

Thirdly, Iridiagnosis provides a vindication of homoeopathic as opposed to allopathic medicine. One of the foundations on which Lindlahr builds his whole theory and system of therapeutics is a belief in the Law of Opposites, the Law of Similars or the Law of Action and Reaction which is a great natural law exhibiting itself in different ways and forms throughout nature, and not least in the human body. It may be stated that when the body is subjected to some particular physical or chemical stimulus it reacts in a particular way and exhibits certain phenomena, but this immediate and short term effect is followed by an opposite and more permanent effect. The classical example which Lindlahr gives of this is in the realm of hydrotherapy where he shows that people who have a sluggish skin which is inefficient as an eliminating and temperature response organ only make it worse by soaking themselves continually in hot baths, as they very often do. For if the first effect of cold water on the body is to produce shivering, goose flesh and a feeling of cold, the longer term effect is to produce a feeling of warmth leading after a time to an improvement of the condition of the skin which reduces the tendency to feel and "catch" cold. In the realm of medication homoeopathy is based on the discovery by Hahnemann that a disease condition can be treated successfully by small doses of a substance which normally gives the same or similar symptoms to that of the disease. If this is sound it is fairly certain and obvious that if medicine is given, as it often is, on the principle of contraries rather than similars, it will tend in the long run to make the condition worse. It is observable that this in fact does very generally happen as, for instance, when constipation is made worse and more chronic by the use of chemical aperients and cathartics. The chapters in the book which deal with the various drugs which are in common use by orthodox doctors are of very great interest because they give in each case the common uses of the drug and its toxological effects, drawn from recognized text books, and this is followed by a description of the signs in the iris which it produces and a note of the way in which it can be expected to be eliminated during natural treatment. There are throughout the book numerous case reports which show how chronic disease has been produced by suppressive treatment of acute disease and how health can be restored by natural treatment. The iridiagnostic findings in these cases are discussed and in many cases illustrated and it is demonstrated how the history, progression and prognosis of a case can be traced in the iris. Needless to say homoeopathic medication does not produce discolourations or other signs in the iris because the preparations, though sometimes based on things which are poisonous in large doses, are so prepared, subdivided, triturated and "potentized" that they act on the body without being retained in it. In fact it appears that in the homoeopathic remedy we are dealing with energies rather than with chemical substance except perhaps in cases where a tincture or a very low potency is being used, and even in these cases the amount is infinitely small. Of special interest to homoeopaths is Lindlahr's discussion of Hahnemann's theory of psora which has sometimes been a stumbling block to homoeopaths. Iridiagnosis provides confirmation of Hahnemann's contentions in this regard by identifying the "itch spots" signs in the iris which are the evidence of psoric suppression.

In conclusion it may be said that Iridiagnosis, if accepted and rightly interpreted, gives absolute proof that disease can be suppressed in various ways of which the use of drugs is the commonest and most important. Substances which are alien and poisonous when retained in the body produce signs in the iris, and this includes elements which are not in themselves alien to the body and may even be essential to its economy, but which are administered in a crude inorganic form. Examples of this are iron and sodium, both of which are essential to the body, but which can do enormous harm if administered in inorganic forms, though common salt does not make any sign in the iris and can be used by the body to a limited extent without causing apparent harm if there is a deficiency of sodium in the soil or in the diet. There is also a considerable difference between drugs in the degree of harm which they do and in the ease or difficulty with which they can be eliminated by the body. It may be said that metallic elements such as mercury and lead are particularly damaging in their effects and particularly hard to eliminate, and such things as arsenic, bromine and quinine are not much better. The drugs which have traditionally been used in the treatment of syphilis are particularly harmful and damaging to the central nervous system and Lindlahr maintains that so-called "tertiary" syphilis is caused by them and not by syphilis. It is probably the elements and substances which are alien to the body in any form which do the most harm and are most difficult to eliminate, but iodine is perhaps an exception to this as it can do great harm and be difficult to eliminate although it is an element of which the body does have need to a certain degree. It is clear that there is need for much more research, observation and study into the whole subject of Iridiagnosis before it can be said to be a complete science and all its possibilities explored. To take one example, a development which has taken place since Lindlahr's time is the discovery and elaboration of antibiotics which are now used to an enormous extent instead of, or in addition to, drugs. This would seem in some ways to be an improvement, but there is little doubt that antiobiotics too are suppressive, at least in the way in which they are now generally used. Whether their use produces changes or signs in the iris is a matter upon which research should no doubt be undertaken if this has not been done already. There is a revival of interest in iridology and homoeopathy and herbalism. Lindlahr's system of treatment was based mainly on dietetics, hydrotherapy and manipulation and he has little to say about herbalism. It has, however, been found that herbalism as well as homoeopathy are of great assistance in bringing about the eliminations and purification of the system which are required in the treatment of chronic conditions and which can be monitored by iridiagnosis during the course of treatment.*

---

*I am informed by a well known iridologist who is also a herbalist that the use of antibiotics does indeed produce signs in the iris, especially in the lymphatic and liver areas. It is claimed by herbalists that certain herbal preparations can be used very successfully in situations where the use of antibiotics is now considered to be advisable or essential.

CHAPTER I

IRIDOLOGY

Correct diagnosis is the first essential to rational treatment. Every honest physician admits that the old school methods of diagnosis are, to say the least, unsatisfactory and uncertain, especially in ascertaining the underlying causes of disease. Therefore we should welcome any and all methods of diagnosis which throw more light on the causes and the nature of disease conditions in the human organism.

Two valuable additions to diagnostic science are now offered to us in Spinal Analysis and the Diagnosis from the Iris of the Eye. Spinal analysis furnishes valuable information concerning the connection between disease conditions and misplacement of vertebrae and other bony structures, contractions or abnormal relaxation of connective tissues, and inflammation of nerves and nerve centres.

Men of high standing in the profession have many times admitted the uncertainty of medical diagnosis, but never has more enlightening information on this subject been furnished than by Dr. Cabot of Harvard University, one of the foremost diagnosticians in this country, and author of a standard work on diagnosis. In a recent address before the American Medical Association he stated that postmortem examinations of one thousand cases which he had conducted disclosed the fact that the antemortem diagnoses were correct in only fifty-three percent of these cases. The following table compiled by Dr. Cabot gives the nature of the various diseases and the exact percentage of correct diagnoses in each.

DISEASE	PERCENT
Diabetes Mellitus	95
Typhoid	92
Aortic Regurgitation	84
Cancer of the Colon	74
Lobar Pneumonia	74
Chronic Glomerulonephritis	74
Cerebral Tumour	73
Tubercular Meningitis	72
Gastric Cancer	72
Mitral Stenosis	69
Brain Haemorrhage	67
Septic Meningitis	64
Aortic Stenosis	61
Phthisis, acute	59
Miliary Tuberculosis	52
Chronic Interstitial Nephritis	50
Thoracic Aneurism	50
Hepatic Cirrhosis	39
Acute Endocarditis	39
Peptic Ulcer	36
Suppurative Nephritis	35
Renal Tuberculosis	33
Bronchopneumonia	33
Vertebral Tuberculosis	23
Chronic Myocarditis	22
Hepatic Abscess	20
Acute Pericarditis	20
Acute Nephritis	16

Dr. Cabot's candid report surely gives food for serious thought. If his colleagues on the staff of the Massachusetts General Hospital, with excellent scientific equipment at their command, failed to render a correct diagnosis in about fifty percent of one thousand cases, what may be expected of the average less skilled physician and surgeon in general practice? Correct prescription, according to allopathic standards, can be based only on correct diagnosis. The old school of medicine recognizes hundreds of different diseases, each one an entity by itself arising from specific causes — mostly disease germs. From this is follows that each specific disease must be treated by specific drugs, vaccines, serums and antitoxins, or by specially devised operations. It is evident that the wrong remedy applied in a given case will not only prove useless, but may cause serious injury; yet if fifty percent of all diagnoses rendered in our best equipped hospitals are erroneous, how can the doctors apply the right remedy? Will somebody please explain?

Compare with this extremely dangerous guess work the safe and sane methods of Natural Therapeutics. Perfectly harmless in themselves, when applied with a modicum of common sense they tend to correct in any case the three primary manifestations of disease. This, I have fully explained in Chapter XX, Vol.I , of this series. While the allopathic physician must postpone the administration of his specific remedies until he gets ready to make a guess — first at the nature of the disease, and then at the indicated remedy — the practitioner of Natural Therapeutics applies his natural remedies with absolute safety, and assurance of success if that is possible in the nature of the case, from the first appearance of abnormal symptoms. Thereby he frequently cures the disease before his allopathic colleague would get ready to treat it. In many cases medical indecision and procrastination allow the disease processes to make such headway that they cannot be arrested by any means.

Dr. Cabot is not the only allopathic physician who admits an appalling discrepancy between clinical findings and the revelations of postmortem examinations. According to a recently published report of a committee appointed to investigate New York hospitals, the autopsies of the famous Bellevue Hospital prove that out of every hundred diagnoses made by the physician in charge 47.7 percent are absolutely wrong. These figures coincide very closely with those of Dr. Cabot. This revelation of medical incompetence caused Dr. C.L. Wheeler, editor of the New York Journal of Medicine, to make the following sensational statement, "Every doctor in America is a quack — and he can't help it. This statement is amazing only to a layman, no doctor is surprised at it. Doctors know that all of us are more or less quacks; that many of our diagnoses are only guess work; and we all know what is far worse than this — that we cannot help it because our hands are tied. Why is this? Because the public refuses medicine the right to become an exact science by objecting to the performance of an autopsy in every case of death." Dr. Wheeler evidently has not learned the lesson taught by these autopsies, namely, that the allopathic conception of the nature of disease and its methods of diagnosis and prognosis as well as of treatment, are all wrong in the first place. He might just as well try to prove that 100 x 0 equals 1 as to establish an exact science of diagnosis by multiplying autopsies. The postmortem examination may reveal the final stages of destruction in vital organs, but medical science will continue to fail in diagnosis and prognosis as long as it does not understand or refuses to understand that such destruction is brought about through wrong habits of living and through unnatural methods of treatment. This is a serious accusation. Why should conscientious physicians refuse to investigate the true nature and causes of disease? The answer is: Because such knowledge comes from "unethical" sources; because from the viewpoint of medical ethics it is better to let a patient die in the "regular" way than to see him cured in the "irregular" way.

Not the opposition of the public to autopsies is responsible for the inadequacy of allopathic diagnosis and prognosis, but the fact that orthodox medicine is not an exact science because it bases its findings on the chaotic and contradictory teachings of medical authorities instead of studying and complying with the laws of nature governing the processes of health, disease and cure. This valuable knowledge is freely offered to the medical profession by the School of Natural Therapeutics. As long as they refuse to give fair consideration to this exact philosophy and science of disease and cure, the teachings of which are verified by the experience of millions of intelligent followers all over the earth and in the daily practice of tens of thousands of drugless healers in this country, they must stand convicted of wilful indifference and neglect. Since prominent members of the medical profession admit the utter inadequacy of allopathic methods of diagnosis and prognosis, why should we hesitate to welcome such valuable aids to diagnostic science as Iridology, Spinal Analysis and Basic Diagnosis, when every one of these helps to elucidate, to correct or to confirm the findings of other methods? Is it not a matter of common sense and personal responsibility towards our patients that we should combine in diagnosis as well as in treatment all that is good and helpful? In the light of these revelations, what reliance can we place on medical health certificates issued to candidates for marriage? What value can be attached to enforced medical examinations in our public schools? What right have medical practitioners to pronounce chronics and defective uncurable, to sterilize them, or to kill them by the refusal of medical aid or by the practice of euthanasia?

Is Iridiagnosis Sufficient to Diagnose Disease?

Iridology is as yet a new science, and much remains to be discovered and to be better explained. Many times we do not find a sign in the iris for the lesion or diseased condition which we know to exist in the body. At other times the records in the eyes indicate more serious conditions than can be ascertained by other methods. As regards this point, however, it is well to remember that old school physicians, notwithstanding their up-to-date scientific equipment, only too often see their diagnosis discredited by the postmortem findings. Thus those who confine their examinations to the eye or the spine fall as far short of making a reliable diagnosis or prognosis as the old school country doctor with his limited equipment. In our work we do not confine ourselves to Iridiagnosis, but combine with it the diagnostic methods (physical diagnosis) of the allopathic school of medicine, spinal analysis, basic diagnosis, as well as laboratory tests and microscopic examinations. Thus any one of these methods supplements and verifies all the others. In this way only is it possible to arrive at a thorough and definite understanding of the patient's condition.

The Story of a Great Discovery

Dr. von Peckzely, of Budapest in Hungary, discovered nature's records in the eye, quite by accident, when a boy ten years of age. Playing one day in the garden at his home, he caught an owl. While struggling with the bird, he broke one of its limbs. Gazing straight into the owl's large, bright eyes, he noticed, at the moment when the bone snapped, the appearance of a black spot in the lower central region of the iris, which area he later found to correspond to the location of the broken leg. The boy put a splint on the broken limb and kept the owl as a pet. As the fracture healed, he noticed that the black spot in the iris became overdrawn by a white film and surrounded by a white border (denoting the formation of scar tissues in the broken bone). This incident made a lasting impression on the mind of the future doctor. It often recurred to him in later years. From further observations he gained the conviction that abnormal physical conditions are portrayed in the eyes.

As a student, von Peckzely became involved in the revolutionary movement of 1848 and was put in prison as an agitator and ringleader. During his confinement he had plenty of time and leisure to pursue his favourite theory, and he became more and more convinced of the importance of his discovery. After his release he entered upon the study of medicine, in order to develop his important discoveries and to confirm them more fully in the operating and dissecting rooms. He had himself enrolled as an intern in the surgical wards of the college hospital. Here he had ample opportunity to observe the eyes of patients before and after accidents and operations, and in that manner he was enabled to elaborate the first accurate Chart of the Eye. Since von Peckzely gave his discoveries to the world, many well known scientists and conscientious observers in Austria, Germany, Sweden and in this country have devoted their lives to the perfection of this wonderful science. Foremost among the followers of von Peckzely in Europe was the Rev. Niels Liljequist, a Swedish clergyman, who, for many years, has made Iridology his life work. He perfected Peckzely's chart of the iris and was the first one to describe the signs of drug poisoning. He had suffered terribly from most of the symptoms of quinine poisoning (chronic cinchonism) ever since he had taken large quantities of the drug in early life. After he became acquainted with iridiagnosis he discovered the connection between the yellow discolouration in his eyes and the chronic quinine poisoning. This led him to study the relationship of other colour pigments to other forms of drug poisoning, such as iodism, mercurialism, bromism, arsenical poisoning etc. In Germany Dr. Thiel and Pastor Felke made valuable contributions to Iridology, and became famous diagnosticians and Nature Cure physicians. In this country Henry Lahn, M.D., wrote the first book in the English language on this new and valuable method of diagnosis. Many years of personal acquaintance with this remarkable man and his work impels me to give him credit for being the ablest iridiagnostician now living. Anderchou in England published a few years ago a brief summary of the discoveries and teachings of the pioneers of Iridology.

The "regular" school of medicine, as a body, has ignored and will ignore this science, because it discloses the fallacy of their favourite theories and practices and because it reveals unmistakably the direful results of chronic drug poisoning and ill advised operations. Leaving out of consideration everything that is at present speculative and uncertain, we are justified in making the following statements, subject to the qualifications and limitations before described:

(1). The eye is not only, as the ancients said, "the mirror of the soul", but it also frequently reveals abnormal conditions and changes in every part and organ of the body.

(2). Organs and parts of the body are represented in the iris of the eye in well defined areas. (See Chart)

(3). The iris of the eye contains an immense number of minute nerve filaments, which through the optic nerves, the optic thalami and the spinal chord are connected with and receive impressions from every nerve in the body.

(4). The nerve filaments, muscle fibres and minute blood vessels in the different areas of the iris reproduce the changing conditions in the corresponding parts or organs.

(5). By means of various marks, signs, abnormal colours, or discolourations of the iris, nature reveals transmitted disease taints and hereditary lesions.

(6). By signs, marks and discolourations, nature also makes known acute and chronic inflammatory or catarrhal conditions, local lesions, destruction of tissues, various drug poisons, and changes in structures and tissues caused by accidental injury or by surgical mutilations. (Figs. 12,28)

(7). The diagnosis from the iris of the eye positively confirms Hahnemann's theory that acute diseases have a constitutional background of hereditary or acquired disease taints or systemic encumbrances.

(8). This science enables the diagnostician to ascertain, from the appearance of the iris, many of the patient's inherited and acquired tendencies toward health and toward disease, his condition in general, and the state of various organs in particular. Reading nature's records in the eye, he can predict many of the healing crises through which the patient will have to pass on the road to health.

(9). The iris frequently reveals dangerous changes in vital parts and organs from their inception, thus enabling the patient to avert threatening disease by natural living and treatment.

(10). Changes in the iris indicate plainly the gradual purification of the system, the elimination of morbid matter and poisons, and the readjustment of the organism to normal conditions under the regenerating influences of natural living and treatment.

How the Signs in the Iris are Produced

The effects of surgical operations performed under anaesthesia either do not show in the eyes at all, or only very faintly, though entire organs or large parts of the body may have been removed by the surgeon's knife. This is due to the fact that under anaesthesia the sensory nerves are benumbed and paralyzed; for this reason we do not feel pain. This condition of temporary paralysis prevents the transmission of impulses to the iris and thereby the production of corresponding signs or lesions in the eye. For instance, the loss of a leg amputated under anaesthesia may not show in the eyes, while the scar tissue caused by the bite of a dog, a wound received from a bullet, or other injury received in the waking, conscious conditions, may show for life in the form of a closed lesion in the iris. These facts prove that the lesions in the eyes are made through abnormal or pathological nerve impulses, which throw the nerve fibres and other structures in the surface layers of the iris out of their normal arrangement. Inflammatory processes incidental to the healing of wounds show temporarily as white signs.

Discolourations or colour signs in the eyes are created by colour pigments carried into and deposited in the surface layers of the iris through the capillary circulation. The dark signs of subacute and chronic catarrhal conditions and of loss of substance or death of tissues are created through atrophy and sloughing of nerve and muscle fibres in the surface of the iris, or depressions and holes in the deeper layers.

I have frequently heard the question, "How is it possible that lesions in the body show in the iris on the same side, when all the afferent nerves cross to the opposite brain half? According to this, lesions in one side of the body should show in the opposite iris." The answer is — the crossing of the optic nerves brings back the signs in the iris to the side of the body in which the corresponding lesion in located. Exceptions to this are lesions in the brain. They cross over in optic nerves, and show in the opposite iris. Thus lesions in the right brain half show in the left iris and vice versa.

CHAPTER II

ANATOMY OF THE IRIS

Since this volume is intended for the use of the layman as well as of the practising physician, I shall endeavour to make the anatomical description as brief and simple as possible. To go into detail would only serve to confuse the layman and would not be of any special advantage to the trained scientist.

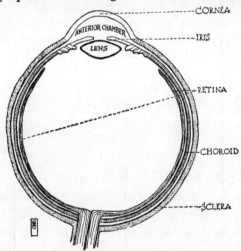

Fig. 1. Cross Section of Eyeball.

The eyeball is a hollow, elastic body, about one inch in diameter and nearly spherical in form. The segment of a smaller sphere projects in the front. The larger sphere is made up of three coats — the sclera, choroid and retina.

1. The sclera or sclerotic coat is a tough, opaque fibrous membrane which surrounds about five-sixths of the eyeball. It serves to protect the inner parts from injury and to preserve the spherical shape of the eye. The cornea is a continuation of the sclera and covers the frontal part of the eye which encloses the anterior chamber containing the aqueous humour. The cornea is as transparent as glass, so as to admit the light unhindered into the interior of the eye.

2. The choroid, or middle coat, is made up of connective tissue, blood vessels and pigment cells. The purpose of the choroid layer and the ciliary body is to supply nutriment to the whole eyeball. The iris is a forward continuation of the choroid coat. It is a circular, mobile, coloured curtain, suspended in the aqueous humour behind the cornea and in front of the crystalline lens. It is perforated a little towards the nasal side of its centre by a circular aperture called the pupil. The iris receives its name (iris, irides — a rainbow) from the varying colour effects.

3. An inner coat, called the retina, which is an extension of the optic nerve, serves to receive impressions from the outside world and conveys them through the optic nerve to the centre of vision in the occipital lobe of the cerebrum.

Structure of the Iris (Fig.2).

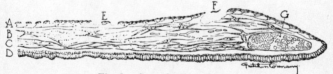

Fig. 2.   Cross Section of Iris.

A. **Surface Endothelium.** This is a single layer of flat endothelial cells continuous with the posterior lining of the cornea.

B. **Stroma.** This is a closely packed mesh-work of delicate radiating connective tissue fibres, enmeshing numerous nerve filaments, blood vessels, lymph vessels and large, irregularly branched connective tissue cells. In the deeper layers of the stroma a band of involuntary muscle fibres,

about 1mm in width, encircles the pupillary margin of the iris.
Reflex contraction of this sphincter diminishes the size of the
pupil. Some authorities describe also radiating muscle fibres
stretching from the border of the sphincter to the circumference of the iris. In all probability, however, these are elastic and not muscle fibres, the dilation of the pupil being
accounted for by the relaxation of the sphincter muscle and
the resulting automatic contraction of the elastic fibres. The
brighter the light, the more contracted the pupil, and vice
versa. This mechanism aims to regulate the amount of light to
be admitted to the retina.

C. **Basement Membrane.** This consists of strong connective
tissue, which forms the support and innermost layer of the
iris.

D. **The pigment layer.** This consists of two rows of epithelial
cells of a dark purple colour, which rest on the uneven surface
of the basement membrane of the iris. This pigment layer serves to prevent the penetration of light through the iris into the
inner dark chamber of the eyeball.

The Normal Colours of the Iris

As described in Chapter IV, there are only two normal iris
colours — light azure blue and light hazel brown. The stroma
of the blue iris is devoid of pigment, thus allowing the purple
pigment layer to shimmer through as a uniform, clear sky
blue. In the normal brown iris the connective tissue cells of
the stroma contain a brown pigment which totally obscures
the purple pigment layer, thus imparting a uniform, clear
light brown colour to the iris. The albino iris contains no pigment either in the connective tissue cells of the stroma or in
the pigment layer. The resulting transparency renders the
blood vessels visible, hence the iris presents a delicate pink
appearance. For the sake of avoiding confusion we will hen-
ceforth consider only the Indo-Caucasian iris which is normally of a uniform brilliant azure colour.

The Blood Supply of the Iris (Fig.3)

The long and short ciliary blood vessels form a complete ring
around the peripheral border of the iris. From this major circle
branches are given out which converge toward the pupil.

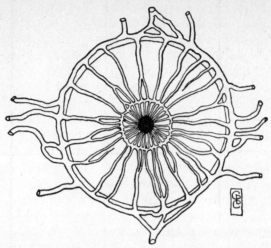

Fig. 3.   Blood Supply to Iris.

At a short distance from the outer border of the sphincter muscle they divide and anastomose to form a second ring. From this minor circle branches continue their course to the pupillary border.

The Nerve Supply of the Iris (Fig.4)

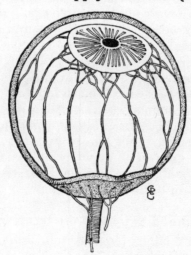

Fig. 4.

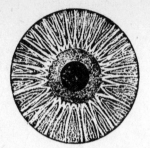 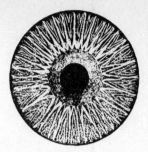

Fig. 4a. Triangles Formed by Nerves.

The nerve supply of the iris deserves special attention. The circular muscle fibres are supplied by the short ciliary nerve branch of the motor occuli, or third cranial nerve, coming directly from the brain. The other structures are supplied by the long ciliary nerve, which is in direct communication with the cervical ganglia of the sympathetic nervous system. These nerves travel forwards to the iris through the choroid coat of the eyeball. Along the attached margin of the iris they form a plexus from which nerve filaments are given off to the muscle fibres and other structures of the iris. Some of these nerve filaments also go to form a complete network on the surface of the iris immediately under the surface endothelium. These are arranged in triangles, the bases of which rest on the outer margin of the iris, and whose apices point toward the pupil (Fig. 4a). The sides of these triangles coincide with the blood vessels, these with the sympathetic nerve supply, and these in turn with the borders of the organ areas. The direct connection of the nerve filaments in the surface layers of the iris with the cervical ganglia of the sympathetic nervous system explains how impressions (vasomotor changes) from all over the body may be conveyed to the iris.

CHAPTER III

EXPLANATION
OF THE KEY TO IRIDOLOGY

Every important part and organ in the body has its corresponding location in the iris in a well defined area, as outlined in the chart. As long as an organ is in normal condition, the corresponding area in the iris presents the normal colour, either light blue or light brown, without any mark, sign or discolouration whatsoever. When an organ or part of the body undergoes acute or chronic changes as a result of hereditary influences, systemic or drug poisoning, or from mechanical injury, then these pathological changes are recorded in the corresponding area of the iris. Pregnancy, though involving profound changes in the organism, is not indicated in the iris because it is a normal physiological process. Surgical mutilations of the body performed under anaesthesia do not show in the iris, or only very faintly, because anaesthesia benumbs and paralyses the sensory nerves and thereby prevents the transmission of nerve impulses to the iris. Any substance congenial to the body, i.e., naturally belonging to it, does not show in the iris. All substances not congenial to the body, i.e., those which do not belong to it, such as minerals and earthy elements in the inorganic form, and all poisons, show in the iris in well defined signs and colour changes in the areas corresponding to the parts or organs where these substances have accumulated.

The arrangement of the areas in the iris is symmetrical

and somewhat in harmony with the locations of the various
parts and organs in the body. We find the area of the stomach
directly around the pupil and the field of the intestines surrounding the region of the stomach. The outer border of the
intestinal field, the "sympathetic wreath", corresponds to the
sympathetic nervous system, and all other parts and organs of
the body radiate from or run into this sympathetic wreath. All
this is in correspondence with conditions in the body. The
stomach and intestines are centrally located, they are to the
body what the fire box is to boiler and engine. The entire
organism is dependent upon the digestive organs for the elements of nutrition and fuel material. Every cell and organ of
the body depends upon the sympathetic nervous system for
its supply of vital energy. All involuntary vital functions and
activities are controlled and directed through the sympathetic
nervous system. This is indicated in the iris by the fact that the
areas of the various parts and organs start or radiate from the
sympathetic wreath. Thus the brain with its divisions, sub-
divisions and special centres is located in the upper regions of
the iris, analagous to the location of the brain in the body. The
distinctly human intellectual faculties, capacities and powers
are located, in right-handed people, in the left brain hemisphere, but reflected through crossing of the optic nerves into
the right iris. In left-handed people the condition is the
reverse. The area of the leg is located in the centre of the lower
half of the iris, etc. Those organs which are located on one

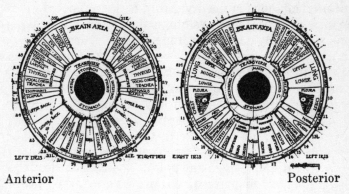

Anterior   Posterior

Fig. 5. Split Circles.

side of the body appear only in the corresponding iris. The heart and spleen, for instance, are represented in the left iris. The corresponding halves of organs divided by the median line of the body, such as the nose, mouth, bladder and genital organs, appear in both irides.

The symmetry of the divisions of the iris is much more real than is apparent on superficial examination. This becomes more clear as we study closely the interdependence of the various parts of the body. The relation between the regions of the iris and the corresponding organs and parts of the body is further illustrated in Fig.5, which is constructed by the following procedure: Divide each iris of the regular key vertically through the centre. Put the outer halves together and imagine the resulting circle to be as large as the body. Then place the resulting large imaginary circle on the anterior aspect of the body in such a way that the pupil covers the umbilicus. Similarly, the circle formed by the apposition of the inner halves is placed on the posterior aspect of the body. By imagining these maps to be vertically and horizontally enlarged so as to cover the entire anterior and posterior aspects of the body, the areas will be found to correspond closely to the different parts of the body. This symmetrical correspondence of the organ areas in the iris to the location of the organs in the body is conclusive evidence that this arrangement is not accidental, but is in harmony with nature's definite design and purpose, and thus amply justifies scientific inquiry into the mysterious cypher language of the iris.

EDITOR'S INTRODUCTION
TO CHAPTER IV

The part of this chapter which discusses the normal or natural colour of the iris presents difficulties to an editor and, after due consideration, I have somewhat abridged and rearranged parts of the original text because I felt it to contain material which was controversial, out of date or irrelevant to the study or iridiagnosis as such. Lindlahr's main point here is to establish that the normal colour of the iris is either light blue or light brown and that eyes become darkened or exhibit other colours only as the result of pathological conditions in the body. He goes on to say that the normal colour of a person's eyes is determined by his racial descent, some races being blue eyed by nature and some brown. Lindlahr had very definite ideas about race and its origins, meaning and implications which he seems to have derived mainly from theosophical sources, though, being himself of German origin, he may have been influenced to some extent by the kind of ideas which, in a perverted form, led to such terrible consequences in Germany in the time of Hitler. Since Lindlahr's time there has been much thought and study devoted to the history and prehistory of man and of the planet, and such sciences as geology, archaeology, palaeontology, biology, anthropology and genetics have made great advances, in the light of which his ideas should be considered and evaluated. It is clear that he intended to clarify and develop his ideas about race and eugenics in Volume V of his series to which he often refers but which was not ever published. However, it would seem that his basic belief was that change and development and evolution of the planet and of its inhabitants are things which are going on continuously. Races, like individuals, are born, become mature, grow old and eventually decay and die. There is an evolutionary process which brings about development of new and more advanced races from those which have gone before. He is very sure that the fifth or "Aryan" root race and particularly its North-European fair and blue eyed sub-races are the most advanced and evolved of the world's races at the present time. He is very much opposed to what he calls "mongrelization" or "miscegenation" especially as between races which are very different in origin and history such as the white, yellow and black races. He also seems to have felt that mankind has now reached a stage where it can and should consciously co-operate with the evolutionary process by healthy living and good mating.

While all these questions and ideas do not have a direct bearing on the science and practice of iridiagnosis as such, and while some of Lindlahr's statements and conclusions on these matters are hard to accept, there is still much of interest and importance in what he has to say and which has a bearing on all sorts of political, social, legal and international questions which will have to be faced in a world which is rapidly becoming a single entity. For example, though too much inbreeding may be bad within small communities, and nations and families may be improved by receiving some admixture of blood from outside, we should, perhaps, on the whole try to concentrate on breeding from our own best and healthiest stocks. Also if there is, or should be, such a thing as eugenics we should seek to have laws and customs which are eugenic and not dysgenic in tendency, without interfering too much with individual liberty and choice. Again, it may be that so called "apartheid" in the original sense of separate development, social life and political institutions may have something to be said for it in the case of races which are very different from each other, provided that it is not based on the oppression or exploitation of one race by another. In this connection it must, surely, be realised that the complete social admixture and free movement and settlement of everybody everywhere would logically lead in time to the whole world being inhabited by a mixed race of some indeterminate beige colour and the probable end of white races which are much less numerous than the others. It must surely be a question of how

far such developments would be to the advantage of mankind
or of the races of which it is composed. It is, perhaps, unfortunate that at the present time it seems virtually impossible
for anyone to discuss the problems arising from race or even
to suggest that race has any real existence or meaning without
being branded a racialist and beyond the pale.

CHAPTER IV

A UNIFORM DIVISION AND CLASSIFICATION OF DISEASE

Students of iridology frequently complain that this interesting science has not been sufficiently systematized for purposes of intelligent study. In order to overcome this difficulty and to facilitate the study, I have divided the successive stages in the development of diseases into four well defined "stages of encumbrance". Such a uniform division and classification of disease conditions and of the corresponding records in the iris, once established, will greatly facilitate the study of Natural Therapeutics and of the diagnosis from the iris. It will also serve to establish a well defined phraseology intelligible to the layman and especially valuable to students and practitioners.

The Four Stages of Encumbrance.

We distinguish in the development of chronic diseases the following four distinct stages of encumbrance:

1. Hereditary and congenital stage.
2. Acute and subacute inflammatory stage.
3. Chronic stage.
4. Chronic destructive stage, accompanied by loss of substance.

All chronic diseases (not caused by violence or conditions uncongenial to human life) which end fatally, pass through four successive stages of encumbrance. Chronic dis-

ease never develops suddenly in the human body. Nature
always tries to prevent its gradual development by acute and
subacute healing efforts. If these, by any means whatever,
are checked and suppressed, then they are followed either by
fatal complications or chronic after effects, the mysterious
"sequelae" of medical science. Thus we find that the unity of
disease as to causes and manifestations, applies to chronic as
well as to acute diseases.

Hereditary and Congenital Stage of Disease

Iridiagnosis settles forever in the affirmative the question at
to whether or not tendencies to disease are hereditary.
Inherited tendencies are recorded in the iris of the eye in three
ways, by colour, density and hereditary lesions. (1) The
colour of the iris indicates whether the vital fluids and tissues
are pure and normal or affected by disease taints and foreign
substances. (2) The density, that is the woof or grain of the
structures composing the iris, gives us information about the
firmness, vitality and general tone of the tissues of the body.
(3) Hereditary and congenital lesions in the form of shady,
grey, usually ovoid or spindle form spots in the iris of the offspring indicate weakness or disease in corresponding organs
or parts of the bodies of the parents. For instance, if the lungs
of the mother were affected by tuberculosis during pregnancy
this may show in the iris of the child in the form of grey or
shady signs or lesions in the areas of the lungs. I say, may
show, because heredity is subject to many modifying influences. This we shall study more fully in the fourth volume of
this series, entitled "Eugenics, or Man-Building on the Physical, Mental and Moral Planes of Being"*.

Under natural management, however, certain organs or
entire bodies, no matter how badly affected by abnormal
heredity, may outgrow entirely the tendency to weakness and
disease. This is the message of great promise of Natural
Therapeutics to those who fear to assume the responsibility
of parenthood on account of weakness and ill health; provided, of course, that the parents prepare themselves, and
that the offspring be treated prenatally in accordance with the
teachings of natural eugenics.

*This volume never in fact appeared, though it was obviously in preparation during
Lindlahr's lifetime.

Colour of the Iris.

First let us consider the colour of the iris. The question arises, is there a normal colour of the iris, and if so, what is it, and what influences will change it and produce abnormal colour effects? The answer to this is as follows: There are two normal colours of the iris — light brown and light blue. These are subject to change through various hereditary and acquired influences. In the previous chapter I have explained how the anatomical structure of the various layers of the iris accounts for the blue and brown colour effects.

The influence of race heridity on the colour of the hair and eyes is an intensely interesting subject, but I cannot discuss it in the confines of this volume. It will be treated more fully in the fourth volume of this series. However, concerning the subject of racial colour I call attention here to a few interesting facts. There is really no black colour of the eyes. As before stated, brown and blue in various shades of lightness and darkness are the only two normal colours of the iris, and these were originally determined by race heredity. According to esoteric history five great root races have come into existence so far on this planet. The third of these was the Lemurian root race which inhabited the continent of Lemuria or Pan, which occupied a large area of what is now the Pacific Ocean. The similarity of geological formations, flora, fauna, and of ethnological characteristics observed on many thousands of islands in the Pacific Ocean which are supposed to have been the mountain peaks of ancient Lemuria, offer strong evidence in favour of the existence of such a continent. The remarkable ruins on the Island of Madagascar, built of immense blocks of stone, are remains of the gigantic architecture of the Lemurian giants, who were probably the prototype of the Cyclops of Greek mythology.

However this may be, the fourth or Atlantean root race is the first one about which we possess authentic knowledge. Its early subraces were the yellow — Chinese and Mongolian — the black skinned African, and the red and copper coloured Atlantean or Turanian branches. All these offshoots of the fourth or Atlantean root race were brown eyed and black haired.

The fifth or Aryan root race developed from the latest
and most perfect offshoots of the Atlantean race. The first
three offshoots of the great Aryan race — the Hindoo, Arabian and Iranian or Persian subraces — underwent a gradual
change from the copper colour of the latest Atlantean races to
the dusky brunette of the most highly developed products of
the Hindoo, Arabian, Persian, Chaldean and Semitic types.
The last two subraces of the Aryan root race, the Celtic and
Indo-Caucasian branches, completed the transition from the
Asiatic brunette to the blonde type. The fourth or Celtic sub-
race emigrated southwestward from the cradle of the Aryan
race in what is now eastern Siberia, conquered the countries
around the Mediterranean, and founded the ancient Greek,
Latin and Iberian civilizations. From Spain Iberian tribes
emigrated into Ireland and Great Britain. The last or fifth sub-
race of the Aryan root race took its course along the northern
slopes of the Caucasus and tarried there for many thousands
of years before it resumed its westward course into what is
now called the continent of Europe. The offshoots of this sub-
race were the Germanic, Gallic, Gaelic, Anglo-Saxon and
Scandinavian tribes, whose outstanding racial characteristics
were tall stature, egg-shaped skull, fair skin, yellow hair and
azure blue iris.

Causes of Change in Racial Characteristics

If the founders of the Persian, Babylonian, Egyptian, Gre-
cian, Roman and Iberian civilizations were of Aryan descent,
it would appear that their descendants have now lost the typical Aryan racial characteristics to a very large extent. This
would seem to be due to the pure stock being adulterated
through admixture with fourth race people. Even in northern
Europe and in America the Aryan stock has been diluted in
various degrees. However, as regards the colour of eyes,
many who appear to have dark eyes are in reality blue eyed
people or their descendants who have turned dark eyed under
the weakening influences of unhealthy living including such
things as food poisoning, foul air, confinement, over-strain,
over-stimulation, luetic diseases, drugging, vaccination,
lymph, serum, and antitoxin therapy. For the colour of the
iris, whether naturally light brown or light blue, can be

changed to darker tints and pigments through encumbrance of the system with waste matter, disease taints and drug poisons, and by the gradual atrophy and death of tissues. Thus, darkening of the natural blue colour of the eyes of descendants of people of pure Germanic, Anglo-Saxon, Celtic or Scandinavian origin into blackish blue, ashy grey, green or brown is always an indication either of an admixture of blood of darker races or of unnatural habits of living and the unnatural treatment of disease. If children of Indo-Caucasian or Celtic origin are born dark eyed, with eyes of blackish blue, green or brown colour, we find that under the influence of natural management as to feeding, bathing, breathing and under the natural treatment of diseases, the colour of the iris grows lighter and gradually returns to the original sky blue. On the other hand, we find that under the influence of unnatural management, after suppression of acute diseases (nature's healing, cleansing efforts), and after vaccination, drug poisoning, antitoxin, lymph and serum treatment, the iris of the infant becomes darker and exhibits various signs, discolourations and pigmentations which we shall consider in detail later on.

To recapitulate — darkening of the iris never takes place simultaneously with improvement, but always with deterioration of health. Lightening and clearing up of the iris never takes place simultaneously with deterioration but always with improvement in health. In seventeen years' practice and close daily observation of changes in the iris, I have never seen an exception to this rule. This is one of the revelations of nature's records in the iris which make iridology an exact science. The changes in colour are the best indication whether or not the methods of living and of treating diseases are in harmony with nature's laws. If acute elimination takes place through certain parts and organs of the body the corresponding areas in the iris often show much lighter in colour than the remaining parts of the eye, indicating that the eliminating parts and organs have become more active and alive and comparatively purer than the rest of the body.

Instances like the following are of common occurrence in our practice. A few years ago we diagnosed in our college class a brown eyed man who had been suffering from childhood with a psoric constitution and from drug poisoning. While the eyes were dark brown, the areas corresponding to the lungs were comparatively blue. I questioned the students about the meaning of this phenomenon, but failing to receive a satisfactory answer I asked the man whether it was not a fact that of late years he had been eliminating from lungs and bronchi a great deal of phlegm and mucus. This he confirmed and told us that his "chronic catarrh" had been a great annoyance to him. He did not understand that this "chronic catarrh" had probably saved his life, and that, thanks to this continuous elimination, the lungs had purified themselves more thoroughly than had other organs of the body. He was physically based. His weakest organs were the kidneys and his intermediate organs, the lungs. Therefore the lungs, sustained by strong digestive organs, had saved the kidneys from destruction. This is explained more fully in "Basic Diagnosis" later in this volume. Luckily for him he had been under homoeopathic treatment, which did not interfere with this form of elimination. Under suppressive treatment by means of quinine, opiates, coal tar products, etc., this cleansing would have been checked and suppressed. Drug poisons would have been added to disease taints and under such unnatural treatment all sorts of complications, or death, would have been the inevitable result. If he had survived, the areas of the lungs instead of being lighter would have been much darker, and would have shown the black signs of chronic catarrh and of loss of substance (caverns in the lungs).

Iris Colour and Climate

The question may be asked at this point, what has climate to do with changes in the colour of eyes and hair? It is quite generally believed that climatic influences have a powerful effect upon racial colour, that sunlight and great heat tend to darken the eyes and hair. This impression has arisen probably because brunette and dark races and nations predominate in the heated zones. As a matter of fact, however, climatic influences change racial characteristics only temporarily and to a slight degree. The descendants of the blue eyed Dutch retain their blond characteristics to this day in the hot African veldt. Remnants of vandal tribes in North Africa are still blue eyed. The Jew, after being acclimatized for many centuries in northern Russia and Scandinavia, is brown eyed and black haired to this day, provided that in his veins runs the pure Semitic blood.*

---

*It should be mentioned that there are, in fact, many Jews who are blond and blue eyed. Some would say that they are strongly represented among the most talented and able of the race. They apper to be mostly those of Mediterranean rather than eastern European origin.

CHAPTER V
DENSITY OF THE IRIS
(Fig.6)

While colour of the iris is indicative of hereditary traits and of the degree of purity or impurity of blood and tissues, density is a measure of that which we call vitality, tone, power of resistance, recuperative power, etc.

Normal Density
Before proceeding with the study of this subject let me explain what is meant by density. When the structures composing the stroma and surface layer of the iris are normally developed and arranged in an orderly manner so that they lie in smooth, even layers, like the fibres in a perfectly woven fabric, and when the layer of endothelial cells covering the surface of the stroma is intact, then the iris is of normal density and presents a surface of crystalline clearness with the beautiful, glossy appearance of topaz or mother-of-pearl. While such an iris is the rule among animals living in freedom, it is nowadays very rarely found in human beings *It is sometimes seen in cats' eyes, but never in dogs, probably because the cat stubbornly adheres to its natural modes of living, while the dog readily adapts himself to the unnatural habits of living of his master and is, therefore, more prone to disease than any other animal excepting man and the hog.

---

* Lindlahr here quotes from a standard work on anatomy as follows:- The surface endothelium is very perishable, being demonstrable only in fresh specimens obtained from young individuals, and usually with much greater difficulty in the human than in the animal iris.

Burton Hendricks, the cancer expert, claims that the lap dogs
of Fifth Avenue are afflicted with cancer as frequently as are
their luxury loving owners.

Defective Density

In an iris of defective density the nerve and muscle fibres in
the surface layer and stroma are unevenly developed and
arranged — some swollen, others shrunken or entirely
obliterated, all crooked, warped and intermingled. In some
areas the fibres are massed into bundles; in others, entirely
displaced so that the darker underlying layers become
revealed, giving the appearance of dark shadings and black
spots. In some instances the displacement is so deep that
actual holes are formed exposing the dark pigment layer. This
is often the case after serious wounds and fractures entailing
great loss of tissues. Such a hole in the iris was the dark spot
in the owl's eye which led the boy Peckzely to the discovery of
this wonderful science of Iridology. An iris of defective density presents in colour as well as in grain and texture, an
uneven, mottled appearance. As every sign, mark or discolouration in the iris stands for some abnormal condition in
the body, it is clear why defective density indicates lowered
vitality and weakened resistance.

We judge the firmness and tensile strength of a piece of
wood, metal or woven fabric by the fineness and smoothness
of grain and fibre. Correspondingly, we recognize in coarse-

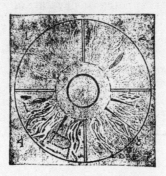

Fig. 6. The Four Densities.

ness, looseness and irregular arrangement of fibre the unmistakable marks of inferiority and lack of tensile strength and stamina. Oak and mahogany have a finer grain than poplar or willow; steel is finer and denser in texture than iron. Similarly, a fine dense iris indicates density and firmness of tissues in the body, and vice versa. In other words, the degree of density of the iris corresponds to the degree of vitality and to the general tone of the system. Since density refers only to the woof of the iris, the scurf rim, medicine signs, lymphatic rosary and itch spots are not taken into consideration in determining the degree of density.

Significance of Density

Since abnormal colour pigments in the iris represent encumbrances of morbid and foreign matter in the system, and since density denotes the degree of integrity and tone of the tissues, colour and density combined indicate the degree of — (a) stamina and endurance, (b) vital resistance to disease, (c) recuperative power and response to treatment, (d) expectancy of life. We judge the quality of the constitution of a person according to the absence or presence in the iris of the various hereditary and acquired taints, encumbrances and defects. The life expectancy of a person can be estimated by the quality of his constitution as revealed in the iris. Frequently however those with frail constitutions carefully nurse their health and outlive those with vigorous constitutions who recklessly squander their vitality.

According to the showing in the iris of colour, density and hereditary lesions, we distinguish four types of constitutions. The ideal, as before stated, we do not find in human beings. We therefore have not given it a place in the drawing (Fig.6.) which illustrates the four degrees of density.

Four Degrees of Density (Fig.6.)

Sections 1. **Good** We notice only a few straight whitish lines. This iris is sometimes found in infants and young children, and in sailors and mountaineers.

Section 2. **Common** The white lines are increased and more tangled. There are a few hereditary lesions and some dark lines indicating subacute, catarrhal conditions; also some nerve rings. Persons exhibiting this degree of density may enjoy good health in the usual sense of the term.

Section 3. **Poor** In this section white lines are more prominent and tangled. It contains several nerve rings. Signs of acute and chronic conditions are more numerous. There are several closed defects. Persons of this type are usually trying one 'cure' after another.

Section 4. **Very poor** In this section signs of chronic and destructive chronic conditions predominate. The nerve rings are partially dark. Closed lesions as in Section 3. Prognosis not promising.

Hereditary and Congenital Lesions

The iris indicates abnormal heredity not only in a general way by darkened colour and defective density, but also in a more definite way by portrayal of hereditary organic defects in the iris of the infant, as produced in Fig.6. Sec.2. In this iris we notice in addition to the whitish lines of acute eliminative activty and nerve rings, signs of organic lesions in the form of ovoid or spindle form shadings. In this manner we have frequently seen weak organs and parts in parents indicated in the iris of the offspring. My eldest son, born when I myself was in a very poor state of health, exhibited by these greyish or hereditary lesions almost every weak part of my own body. Thus the diagnosis from the iris of the eye assists in solving definitely one of the mooted questions of science — that of heredity. All shades and grades of opinion prevail, some authorities claim that there is nothing in heredity; others that weakened resistance only is hereditary; and still others maintain that organic weakness and defects of certain parts and organs may be transmitted to the offspring. That the last are in the right is conclusively demonstrated by iridiagnosis.

Under natural management of nature's acute eliminative efforts, such as skin eruptions, diarrhoeas, fevers, catarrhal conditions, etc., the signs of hereditary and congenital organic defects gradually disappear from the iris of the infant. Under adverse management, however, they deepen and darken into chronic signs. The totality of these various hereditary, congenital, acute, chronic and destructive defects in the iris thus determine the degree of density and serve as a measure of the vitality and recuperative powers of the organism; for it stands to reason that the more seriously vital parts and organs are effected, the lower must be the recuperative power of the entire organism.

It now becomes clear what we meant by our words of solace to the dark eyed folk in the previous chapter. We see now that colour alone does not determine the state of health, vitality or expectancy of life. Brown eyes by virtue of racial descent are normal and not indicative of disease. A person dark eyed as a result of physical abnormality but with an iris of good or common density may enjoy much better health and may have better expectancy of life than a blue eyed person with a density of the fourth grade, indicating serious catarrhal and destructive defects in vital parts and organs. The question may be asked, "Is not this contradictory? You state that the colour of the iris darkens with deterioration in health, and consequently people with defective iris density should always have dark coloured eyes." I would answer to this that under certain influences destruction of vital parts may proceed much faster than the darkening of the colour, but the latter always to some extent accompanies the former. Is it not a matter of common occurence to see blue eyed athletes and prize fighters endowed with magnificent physique and exuberant vitality fall victims to destructive wasting diseases in a few years' time under the influence of riotous living and destructive habits? Colour, density and hereditary defects together are, therefore, the indicators of hereditary, congenital and acquired tendencies toward health and disease.

The Signs of the Second, or Acute Inflammatory Stage of Encumbrance.
Fig.14, Series I, and Fig.10.

From the very commencement of individual life, nature endeavours to purify the infant body of its hereditary disease taints and morbid encumbrances, through acute eliminative processes such as skin eruptions, purgings, acute catarrhal eliminations in the form of coughs and mucous discharges from the nasal passages and other cavities of the body, and through various acute febrile diseases of childhood, such as measles, chickenpox, scarlet fever, etc. The universality of these acute diseases of infancy indicates their hereditary origin. If these eliminative efforts of nature are not suppressed but are encouraged through natural management and treatment, then the little body will purify itself in course of time from hereditary and acquired encumbrances. The length of time required to accomplish this depends upon the nature of the morbid encumbrances and upon the degree of vitality and power of reaction. It may continue for a few months or a few years, or in serious cases the final purifying and healing crises may not develop until the sixth — the first crisis year in the life of a child. These eliminative processes show in the iris of the newborn infant and growing child in the form of a white star which proceeds from the pupil outward in all directions, especially in those organs where elimination is most active, as, for instance, in the digestive tract and respiratory organs (Fig.10). The outer parts of the iris, outside of the white star, are usually of a dark violet, blackish blue or dark brown colour, from which stands forth the white star around the pupil, which signifies acute forms of elimination, such as purging, skin eruptions, catarrhal discharges, febrile diseases, etc.

As the system becomes purified and more normal the iris will approach more and more to the normal light blue or light brown colour, according to the racial descent of the child. If, on the other hand, nature's acute eliminative efforts are checked or suppressed by wrong or, as we call it, unnatural treatment, then the iris assumes a still darker hue and condenses in the outer circumference, where the blue or brown borders on the white cornea, in a dark ring or wreath. This was called by the first iridologists "the scurf rim", because it makes its appearance after the suppression of "milk scurf" and other forms of cutaneous elimination. The formation of the scurf rim marks the beginning of the third or chronic stage of encumbrance and will be described under that heading.

How the White Signs of Acute Inflammatory Lesions are formed in the Iris.

As before stated, all acute inflammatory and febrile conditions in the body are portrayed in the iris by white lines, streaks and clouds. When the entire organism is in a feverish condition, the eyes present the whitish, glistening appearance commonly noticed in high fevers and in states of great mental or nervous strain. Such states of physical and mental excitement accelerate the circulation and produce in the affected parts congestion, swelling and pain. Every acute inflammatory or febrile process is the result of a cleansing and healing effort of nature, the white clouds in the eyes indicate where nature's healing forces, the "vis medicatrix naturae", are at work. When acute inflammation runs its natural course through the five stages, then perfect absorption and reconstruction take place in the affected organ and the resulting condition is better than before the house cleaning. As the inflamed part or organ returns to normal, the white signs of inflammation disappear (Fig.14, Series I,e).

The white signs of acute inflammatory conditions are pro duced anatomically in the following manner: Congestion in any organ or part of the body reflexly gives rise to similar vaso-motor changes in the corresponding organ area in the iris. The congestion in the stroma of the affected area presses the top layers above the level of the surface. The nerve and muscle fibres thus protruding above the surface (being colourless) appear as white wavy lines which when grouped closely together resemble white streaks or clouds. When the congestion and swelling in the middle layers of the iris subside the nerve and muscle fibres of the top layer fall back into their normal positions, and then the surface of the iris resumes its normal blue or brown appearance. When, through injury or surgical treatment, muscular or other tissues have been torn, cut or broken crosswise, the corresponding lesions in the iris run diagonally or crosswise to the surface filaments of the iris, while lesions caused by internal inflammatory processes run parallel with the fibres of the iris. Lesions caused by various injuries are portrayed in Fig.18R, area 17 and Fig.28L, area 18.

The Signs of Subacute Inflamation

Suppose that nature's healing and cleansing efforts are checked or suppressed by various means, such as exposure to wet and cold, lowered vitality, nerve exhaustion, or by ice packs, drugs or surgical treatment, then the acute eliminative pro-

cess enters upon the stages of subacute and chronic destruction of cells and tissues. Let us take for example a case of
acute catarrh of the bronchi and lungs which, under suppressive treatment, gradually enters upon the subacute and
then upon the chronic stages of disease. All drugs which are
usually the working principle in cough and catarrh remedies,
lower the fever and "cure" the catarrh because they are
astringents, opiates and protoplasmic poisons; because they
contract and throttle the secreting cells, benumb and kill the
red corpuscles, paralyze the respiratory centres and heart
action — in short, because they suppress nature's acute healing efforts by lowering the vitality and paralysing the vital
functions. The pathological changes from the acute to the
subacute stages are accompanied by atrophy and sloughing of
cells and tissues, and these are portrayed in the iris by atrophy
of structures in the corresponding organ areas. This produces
the grey and dark shades of "subacute lesions".

The Signs of the Third and Fourth Stages
of Encumbrance.
(Fig.14, Series III)

When by suppressive treatment above described, the secreting cells of the bronchi are hindered in their labours, the
elimination of mucus and pus is suppressed and the debris
resulting from nature's purifying processes is retained in the
cells and tissues of the lungs, drug poisons are added to the
disease poisons and these morbid accumulations become a
source of continuous irritation. While the previous (acute)
violent coughing and expectoration has subsided, there is
now a low, hacking cough; mucus accumulates in the bronchi
during the night and is evacuated in the morning with great
effort. Retention of morbid matter and lowered vitality
gradually cause decay and destruction of lung tissue. These
degenerative processes repeat themselves in slightly mod-
ified degrees in all chronic destructive diseases affecting
other parts and organs. Simultaneously with this destruction
of tissue in the lungs, similar changes take place in the corresponding areas of the iris. In these fields of the iris the tissues
lose their vitality, dry, shrivel and turn dark. As a result of

this the white clouds of acute inflamatory lesions become intermingled with dark shades and streaks, as represented in Fig.14, Series III. When examined with a strong magnifying glass it will be noticed that these dark areas are more or less depressed. In the advanced stages of destruction they deepen into holes, sometimes down to the black pigment layer.

Closed Lesions.
(Fig.14, Series III c and f, Series II, g)

If, under the adverse circumstances above described, nature still succeeds, in an imperfect way, in healing the defects of the lungs or any other part of the body by the formation of scar tissue, the dark signs in the iris become circumscribed by and interwoven with white lines. The more perfect the healing, the more white lines are interwoven with the dark and the more solid the white enclosures. These closed lesions correspond to the scar tissue in the body. At best they indicate weak spots in the system which under certain provocations may at any time again open and become acute, subacute or chronic lesions.

The Signs of the Fourth or Chronic Destructive Stage of Disease.
(Fig.14, Series IV)

The last destructive stages of disease are marked by increasing atrophy and destruction of cells and tissues. When these degenerative changes take place in vital organs the chances of recovery become more and more precarious. In the iris the dark shadings of the subacute and chronic stages become more intensified and change into black shades or spots. Caverns in the lungs, for instance, appear frequently as small black dots in the lung areas of the iris (Fig.27, area 9, left).

The Signs in the Iris of Acute, Subacute and Chronic Disease Processes.
(Fig.14.)

Series I represents the signs of acute inflamatory processes in various stages and degrees of intensity. Acute disease in the stages of greatest intensity — aggravation and destruction — shows in the corresponding organ areas as represented in

Figures a, d and f. As the inflammatory process declines
under natural treatment during the stages of absorption and
reconstruction, the protruding fibres which cause the white
signs fall back into their normal positions and the white lines
or clouds gradually disappear, as presented in Figures g, e and
b. Figure c is a closed lesion in process of formation. We
observe such lesions after pneumonia, pleurisy, nephritis or
any other acute disease which has been suppressed by ice or
drugs. They stand for scar tissue. Under adverse conditions
they may become acute again in a destructive way. Under
natural living and treatment they may become acute (in healing crises) in a constructive way. Closed lesions of long standing and of a chronic nature show as represented in Series II
Figs.g and Series III Figs.c and f.

The Figures in Series II represent inflammatory processes in the subacute stages. These are transitory between
the acute and chronic stages, as explained above. Disease in
the subacute stage yields readily to natural methods of living
and of treatment. The figures from a to f portray lesions of
increasing severity.

The Figures in Series III represent the signs of chronic
catarrhal conditions. The preponderance of black over white
indicates destruction and sloughing of tissues.

The Figures a, b, d and e of Series IV represent the
chronic inflammatory processes in the last destructive stages,
entailing loss of substance. We meet with such signs only in
people endowed with exceptionally robust constitutions.
Most chronic patients succumb when the disease reaches the
stages represented by the lesions shown in Series III. Figures
c and f in Series IV are signs of cancer in the last stage. Sign f
showed very plainly in the iris of a woman dying with cancer
of the stomach. The black spot was located near the pupil.
The white streamers extended to the margin of the iris. We
found lesions c in the intestinal area of a patient suffering
from cancer in the transverse colon.

The Lymphatic Rosary
(Colour Plate, Fig.c. Also Fig.13 and Fig.22)
One of the most interesting signs of the third and fourth stages
of disease is the lymphatic or typhoid rosary. I have given it

this name because the sign appears in the form of white flakes in the outer rim of the iris, resembling the beads of a rosary. This circular area is marked on the chart of the iris "Lymphatic system" (see chart). Wherever the white flakes appear in this area they indicate inflammation and an engorged condition of the lymph nodes in the corresponding parts of the lymphatic system or, in the later stages, an atrophic condition of the lymphatic glands. Frequently we find the flakes discoloured with the characteristic pigments of drug poisons.

Distinction Between Lymphatic Rosary and the Sign of Arsenic.

The lymphatic rosary is not, as Liljequist says, the sign of arsenic, but since arsenic has a special affinity for the spleen and lymphatic system, the engorged condition of the lymph nodes and atrophy of the lymphatic glands may be and undoubtedly is in many cases the result of arsenical poisoning. The poison itself shows in white flakes resembling the beaten white of egg or snow flakes in the outer margin of the iris, therefore they may be easily mistaken for the lymphatic rosary (Colour Plate, fig.b, p). The latter, however, appears only in the outermost rim of the iris, just inside the scurf rim, in orderly arrangement like the beads of a rosary, while the white flakes of arsenic may appear singly or in irregular groups anywhere in the outer half of the iris. We speak of the "typhoid" rosary because in many instances we find the sign in the eyes of people who have suffered from typhoid fever, which on account of suppressive treatment by drugs or ice was not allowed to run its natural course and left the glandular structures of the intestines and of the system in general in a more or less engorged and atrophic condition. This explains why we find the typhoid rosary usually associated with pronounced malassimilation, malnutrition and with the last stages of destructive wasting diseases. Such patients never fully recover from the effects of the disease and only too often drift into tuberculosis, pernicious anaemia or other slow but fatal wasting disease. When under natural treatment the inflammation in the intestines runs its natural course, and when during the last stages of inflammation sufficient time is allowed for the reconstruction of the intestinal membranes and glandular structures, recovery is rapid and complete and the typhoid rosary does not appear in the iris. We find the rosary usually in the lower parts of the iris and as high up as the areas of lungs and neck (Figs.13 and 22), less frequently in the fields of the sensory organs or in the brain region.

Radii Solaris

These signs in the iris must not be mistaken for lesions. They are straight brown or black lines tapering to a fine point, radiating from the pupil or the sympathetic wreath to the outer margin of the iris. We find them most frequently in brown eyes, only rarely in blue. They are probably formed by a massing of dark colour pigment on the surface of the iris. Iridologists have not been able to attach any special significance to these interesting signs. I have found in many instances that they disappeared with general improvement and the clearing up of the brown colour of the iris. Radii solaris are visible in Fig.6, Sections 3 and 4. They are very plain in Fig.9 and Fig.10.

In this connection it may be well to call attention to other conditions in the iris which might be mistaken for signs of lesions. In brown eyes. sometimes the blue underground shows in places through the brown surface. This indicates a good condition of the corresponding organs. In other instances the underlying blue or light brown shows dark in contrast with surrounding light or yellowish discolourations, and may thus be mistaken for dark lesions.

CHAPTER VI

NERVE RINGS
(Figs 7 and 25. Colour plate, c, d, e,f.)

In addition to the white signs, nature also portrays acute healing activity by white nerve rings and by the appearance of the white sympathetic wreath. Nerve rings are concentric rings shown in Fig.7. They look in the iris as though they had been drawn with a white pencil. According to anatomists who have made a special study of the structure of the iris, these rings originate in the following manner: "During the dilation of the pupil the anterior layers of the iris are disposed in folds, the depressions between which constitute the so called "contraction grooves or furrows". The grooves are deepened when the iris narrows and are almost entirely obliterated by being smoothed out as the iris broadens (pupil contracts)." Fig.8, (B-B), shows the contraction grooves as portrayed in standard works of anatomy.

While it may be true, as anatomy claims, that the grooves in the iris are caused by mechanical contractions and dilations of the iris curtain, we claim that these fluctuations in the size of the pupil are also brought about by an over irritated nervous system, by pain, emotional states, etc. This explains why nerve rings appear and disappear in the iris in strict correspondence with pathological conditions in the nervous system. At first they appear white (acute) on account of the fact that all pathological changes occur first in the acute form. (Colour plate, e).

White nerve rings indicate an irritated, over stimulated condition of the central nervous system or of certain parts of it. If they show in certain confined parts or organs only, they often indicate the approach or present activity of healing crises. When they appear in the brain region they indicate a disturbed, irritated or over stimulated condition of brain matter. This is usually accompanied by a nervous mental condition and insomnia (Fig.26.). This nerve irritation, when long continued, produces a benumbed, semi-paralyzed condition of the nerves. These progressive atrophic conditions are portrayed in the iris by the gradual darkening and final blackening of the nerve rings. (Fig.6, Secs.3-4. Colour plate, f.). When the nerve rings appear dark grey or black it means that the corresponding portions of the nervous system have passed from the acute, over irritated condition to the atonic or semiatrophic.

To illustrate — white nerve rings in bronchi and lungs might indicate acute bronchitis or pneumonia. White nerve rings in the brain might indicate hyperactivity, great irritability, hysteria and insomnia through irritation by systemic or drug poisons or by mental or emotional stress. Black nerve rings in the same area would indicate a benumbed or semi-paralyzed condition of brain matter, characterized by great weakness and prostration, loss of memory, numbness and partial paralysis of nervous and mental functions. It is most interesting to observe the gradual change of black nerve rings into white, and in time the entire disappearance of the white rings under natural methods of living and treatment. I have seen the black nerve rings in the iris of many people afflicted with chronic insomnia or with serious mental diseases. As such cases yielded to natural treatment the black nerve rings always changed into white and finally disappeared entirely from the brain region.

The Seven Zones of the Iris

Iridologists so far have, in the worst cases of nerve derangement, discovered only four fully developed nerve rings (Fig.7.). These four nerve rings, from the pupil outward, form five consecutive zones. Imagine the iris divided lengthwise and the nerve rings straightened out and you will have the five zones as in zone therapy for each half of the body. If we count the areas of stomach and bowels as one zone each, and add

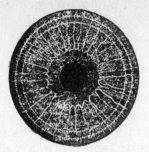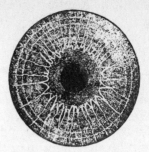

Fig. 7. Concentric Nerve Rings.

them to the five outer zones, then we have again the mystical number seven. Furthermore we find the various organs centre in one or several of these zones; thus the stomach is located in the first zone when we count from the pupil outward, the intestines in the second zone, the pancreas, kidneys and heart in the third zone, the respiratory organs in the fourth zone, and so forth, as outlined in Fig.7a.

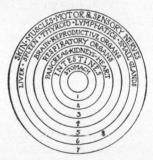

Fig. 7a. The Zones as Determined by the Five Nerve Rings, the Sympathetic Wreath and the Division Between Stomach and Intestine.

Sympathetic Wreath
(See Chart and Figs.8,11,27)

According to Jackson's Anatomy, "the surface radial ridges coming from the edge of the pupil and those radiating from the periphery of the iris, meet in a zig-zag elevated ridge concentric with the pupil called the "corona irides"." This elevated ridge is identical with the area of the sympathetic nervous system in the iris. "Since this ridge corresponds to the situation of the blood vessels of the stroma, the corona irides represents the location of the minor circle" (of blood vessels. (Fig.3.). From the Nature Cure viewpoint, the manifestations of disease occur as vasomotor changes, which are controlled by the sympathetic nervous system. This explains why the blood vessels in the iris and the "sympathetic wreath" are identical in location.

Since the sympathetic wreath forms the outer boundary of the intestinal zone, its widening and branching correspond to a flabby, flacid, atonic, dilated condition of the intestines. Such a relaxed condition of the intestines results in constipation owing to the fact that the musculature of the intestinal walls is too weak to contract on and to propel the food residue (enfeebled peristalsis) (Fig.19.). From this it is plain that in such a condition enemas are particularly contra-indicated, because the habitual injection of warm water still further dilates the already weakened intestinal walls. The indicated spinal manipulation (aside from correcting specific lesions) is to treat the reflex centre in the spine which contracts the intestines — i.e. the second lumbar.

On the other hand, a small narrowed sympathetic wreath signifies a correspondingly spastic, over-irritated condition of the intestines. This brings about spastic constipation with straining at the stool. The indicated spinal treatment in such a case is diametrically opposed to the treatment for the relaxed condition, i.e. stimulate the centre (the eleventh dorsal), which dilates the intestinal musculature.

Osteopaths, chiropractors and naprapaths are sometimes at a loss to account for the fact that in some cases of constipation the patient may immediately respond to adjustment, whereas in other cases the patient apparently gets worse until the spinal lesion has been corrected. To illustrate: Suppose in a case of flaccid constipation where the iris shows a widened sympathetic wreath and the physical examination shows a distended condition of the bowels with gas formation, the spinal lesion happens to be at the second lumbar (the reflex from which centre contracts the intestines), adjustment will not only tend to correct the mechanical lesion but will also elicit nerve reflexes which contract the distended bowel wall. In such cases improvement is noticed long before the spinal lesion is corrected. To illustrate the opposite condition: A

patient with spastic constipation has a spinal lesion in the
second lumbar. In this case adjustments on account of the
reflexes of contraction which they elicit will temporarily
aggravate the condition — spastic constipation — until the
lesion is corrected. In order to prevent these temporary
aggravations, adjustments in this case should be followed by
treatment of the eleventh dorsal so as to dilate the intestines.

We find the contracted sympathetic wreath and 'pinhead' pupil in many types of paralysis, while the distended,
highly mobile pupil is indicative of nervous irritation and
hyper-sensitiveness, as caused, for instance, by intestinal
parasites in children

The Significance of Black and White in the Eye
Symbolism has always identified white with the constructive
principle in nature and black with the destructive principle.
White are the angels of light, black the demons of darkness.
White is the emblem of youth, joy, peace and happiness;
black symbolises old age, war, death, destruction and mourn-
ing. In her picture language in the iris, nature conforms and
upholds humanity's instinctive perceptions. She paints all
constructive processes in white and destructive processes in
black. In this way she confirms the fundamental law of cure
—all acute reactions are the result of nature's healing
efforts.

White Signs the Heralds of Healing Crises
When chronic and destructive processes in the body have
painted in the iris the dark shades and black signs of destruction or loss of substance and the patient has been "given up"
by allopathic practitioners as incurable, when as a last resort
he has adopted natural methods of healing and is approaching
the crisis periods — then the white signs of acute activity in
the dark regions of the iris are as welcome to the sight of the
natural therapist as the white flag of surrender on the fortress
wall to the besieging army. Thus the white signs in the iris, as
well as the white nerve rings, are not only indicators of acute
disease but in chronic cases they become the heralds of
approaching healing crises.

Hippocrates, the father of medicine, said two thousand years ago that it was "the duty of the physician to foresee these changes, to assist and not to hinder them", so that "the sick man might conquer the disease with the help of the physician". The time at which crises were to be expected were naturally looked for with anxiety, and it was a cardinal point in the Hippocratic system to foretell them with precision. With the limited knowledge of diagnostic science at the command of the disciples of Hippocrates this was an exceedingly difficult task. Iridiagnosis not only proves the truth of the teachings of the great master of medicine, but also makes it comparatively easy to carry out his injunction, to foretell and describe the coming healing crises.

The manager of a great sanatorium in this country, scouting the idea of healing crises, says in one of his works that some "tyros" in the art of healing say a great deal about healing crises, but that the violent reactions which they produce are merely the results of harsh treatment. I have treated and cured many patients who were discharged from this and other sanatoriums during the first six weeks of improvement because the doctors in such institutions were under the mistaken impression that the first improvement was a cure, but in many instances these "cured"ones hardly reached home when healing crises made their apparance. Not understanding the meaning of these reactions, the patients were frightened back to the "flesh-pots of Egypt" and to the pills of Dr. Dopem. I have found that others who remained in these institutions during the first improvement until the crisis period, not having been instructed or warned about the significance of these natural reactions, became greatly alarmed, packed their trunks and secretly left for home, believing more firmly than ever in the efficacy of drugs and the surgeon's knife. The following may serve as a typical example.

Some time ago an elderly woman visited a sister who was under our care and treatment. The visitor kindly volunteered the information that she had undergone "this kind of treatment, but that it had done her no good". When questioned about her experience she said that for many years she had suffered from "bowel trouble" and that her family physician had recommended an operation for appendicitis. Dread-

ing the operation, she went instead to a renowned sanitarium
supposed to be working along natural lines of healing. For a
few months her improvement was remarkable, but then all at
once the old pains and inflammations returned. She concluded that the "drugless treatment" was not the thing for her,
returned to Chicago and at once had the offending appendix
removed. "Since that time" she added defiantly, "it has never
troubled me any more". Looking at her enlarged finger joints,
I remarked "Since the operation you have been badly constipated'. "Yes, that is so". "Since that time you have also suffered a great deal of rheumatism". This she also confirmed. I
then endeavoured to explain to her that the removal of the
appendix simply aggravated chronic constipation; that this in
turn was the cause of the rheumatism; that it would have been
better for her if she had stayed in the sanitarium, weathered
the crises and had then been cured permanently of her intestinal ailments. This would have meant restoration of perfect
function, normal action of bowels and kidneys, and freedom
from rheumatism. These suggestions she vehemently resen-
ted. She knew her appendix was "cured" and the rheumatism
had nothing to do with it. Her doctor had told her "the
rheumatiz was caused by the damp Chicago climate". An old
proverb says "Against stupidity even the gods battle in vain".
I left her to enjoy in peace her chronic constipation and her
"rheumatiz". If the doctors in the great sanitarium had
understood the laws of crises, they could have saved, in this
one as well as in many other cases, the reputation of their
institution and of natural treatment — as well as the appendix
of the patient; and they could have spared her a great deal of
chronic suffering. It would have been impossible for me to
hold one half of my chronic patients through the trying times
of acute reaction if I had not been able, from the records in the
iris, to foretell and to describe the future healing crises.

CHAPTER VII

THE SCURF RIM
Figs 8 and 18.

The name Scurf Rim was applied by the first Iridologist to the dark ring often visible in the outer iris of the eye, because it usually appears and is always intensified after suppression of milk crust, scurf, sycotic and other eczematuous eruptions on the heads and bodies of infants and children. The outer rim of the iris, where the iris colour joins the white of the eyeball (sclera) corresponds in the body to the cutaneous surface, the skin. If the skin is normal, healthy and active, the rim of the iris shows no abnormal discolourations. If, however, the skin is weak, enervated, atonic, or in an anaemic and atrophic condition, there appears in the rim of the iris the dark scurf rim. Sometimes this dark ring is complete all around the iris (Fig.18.), sometimes it appears only in certain portions or segments of it (Fig.9.). Suppression of skin eruptions, mercurial inunctions, hot bathing, steam baths, heavy, dense clothing, coddling, or anything else which weakens skin action, tends to intensify the scurf rim.

Hereditary disease, as we have learned in former articles, is indicated in the iris of infants by a general darkening of colour. Sometimes, however, in the offspring of scrofulous, psoric or mercurial parents the scurf rim also is, shortly after birth, more or less distinctly visible. Nature endeavours to purify the tender, plastic body of its hereditary taints and acquired morbid encumbrances, not only through the natural channels of elimination, but also by the various

forms of acute infantile diseases, such as diarrhoeas, skin
eruptions, colds, catarrhs, febrile diseases, etc. Nature's
favourite means of purifying the infant organism are skin
eruptions on head and body. If these are suppressed by
salves, drugs, drying powders, oils, creams, soaps, warm
bathing, warm, dense clothing, and coddling, the scurf rim
appears, or, if already present, becomes more prominent,
indicating that skin action has been weakened and paralyzed
by such unnatural treatment (Fig. 18.). It would probably be
going too far to attribute the scurf rim always to suppression.
As before intimated, the dark rim may be the sign of a weak
and inactive skin not virile enough to produce eruptions.
Such a person, however, has but few chances to survive in the
battle of life, and usually succumbs to the first serious disease
crisis. On the other hand, it is very interesting to observe how
the scurf rim diminishes and gradually disappears when,
under the influence of natural diet, warm sun and light baths,
cold water treatment, massage, neurotherapy, etc., the cuticle becomes alive and active, and through skin eruptions,
furuncles, carbuncles etc., throws off the latent chronic
taints.

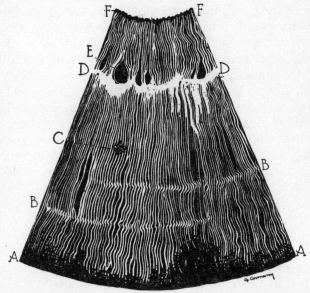

Fig. 8. Section of Iris.

The scurf rim is, therefore, a reliable indicator of the normal or abnormal condition of the skin. This becomes of eminent importance in diagnosis and prognosis when we consider how necessary is normal activity of the skin to the maintenance of health and to life itself. This is due to the fact that the skin, besides containing the superficial organs of touch, has two very important functions — heat radiation and excretion. Our temperature constantly stands near 99 degrees F., no matter whether we are at the equator or in the polar regions; whether we swelter in the heat of summer or shiver in the cold of winter. Deviations of a few degrees either way from the normal heat are symptoms of severe illness. The body is able to maintain this equality of temperature only by the instrumentality of the lungs and of the skin. If the skin is clogged, sluggish, tense or atrophied, then inner blood pressure and temperature rise too high. If the skin is too weak or relaxed, then the loss by radiation is too great and as a consequence inner blood pressure and temperature sink too low. If heat radiation is interfered with, as in high fevers, through uric acid or pathogen poisoning, or through atrophy and clogging of the skin, there results in the interior organs a tendency to congestion, high blood pressure, catarrhal, feverish and inflammatory conditions, which may cause coma and death.

It will be of interest here to study the elimination of morbid matter from the human body as it takes place through the organs of depuration. The principal waste produce of carbohydrate metabolism is CO^2 — carbon dioxide; of protein metabolism $CO(NH^2)^2$ — urea. Imperfect oxidation of carbohydrates and protein matter may result in the formation of many kinds of acids and ptomaines. These must be neutralized and eliminated in the form of salts. The various organs eliminate normally only the following waste products:

Kidneys	Lungs	Skin	Bowels
$NaCO_2$ Large amounts of urea, salts water	Large amounts of CO_2 Trace of salts. Variable amounts of water. No urea.	Small amounts of CO_2. No urea. Considerable amounts of salts — one third of amount of salts eliminated through the kidneys. Considerable amounts of water.	Indigestible and undigested foods, and other waste and morbid products. The latter particularly through the various forms of diarrhoea

When the system is in an abnormal or diseased condition, encumbered with large amounts of waste and morbid matter, then the excretory organs will eliminate many other kinds of waste and morbid materials besides the normal products of excretion mentioned in the foregoing diagram — as, for instance, uric acid and indican in the urine, etc. However, it will be noticed that, normally, the various excretory products are few and simple in form. It is the function of microorganisms, including microzymes, bacteria and parasites, to reduce the highly complex acids, ptomaines, leukomaines and xanthines of normal and abnormal metabolism into simple compounds suitable for elimination through the excretory organs. In this connection I refer the reader to the pathogenic theory of inflammation, Volume I, Chapter IX, according to which inflammation is an effort of nature to reduce or oxidise through bacterial action highly complex albuminous waste (pathogen) into simpler forms more easily eliminated.

The healthy skin excretes considerable amounts of carbon dioxide and numerous other systemic poisons in the form of gases and salts. It does, therefore, a large amount of vicarious work for lungs and kidneys. If the action of the skin is inhibited by sudden chilling, pathogenic obstruction or by other enervating, paralyzing influences, then the internal organs of elimination, in addition to their own, have to do the work of the skin and become congested and overworked, a condition which results in acute catarrhal elimination. That is, the internal membranous linings endeavour to eliminate the pathogenic materials in the form of mucous excretion. But the most important function of the skin, on which depends life itself, is that of heat radiation in connection with the heat regulating centres in the medulla and probably in the pituitary gland. If by burns, scalds or other causes one fourth of the cutaneous surface has become inactive or is destroyed, death is the inevitable result.

We can now understand why the scurf rim, in a measure, stands for what we call the scrofulous constitution because it betokens an inactive, weakened circulation, pathogenic encumbrances, cold extremities, pale, clammy skin and therefore a tendency to chronic catarrhal conditions, all of which prepare the congenial soil for tuberculosis in later life. This brings out in full relief the immense importance in the cure of diseases of the nude air, sun and light baths, cold water treatment, massage, neurotherapy, of porous or no underwear, light clothing, nude sleeping, out of door sleeping, etc. Heavy, dense clothing alone is sufficient to enervate and suppress the natural eliminative activity of the skin, because it prevents free ventilation and keeps the body bathed all day and night in its own poisonous exhalations. This causes and aggravates a multitude of catarrhal ailments and acid diseases.

Often we hear remarks like the following: "I cannot understand why my face is full of blotches, pimples and eruptions when my body is perfectly pure and clean". There is no mystery to this very common phenomenon. The face in such cases has to do the work for the rest of the cutaneous surface because coming in contact with light, air, rain and cold, the face is covered by the only piece of skin on the body which is healthy and capable of active elimination. If these blemished ones would expose their bodies as freely as their hands and face to the health-giving, stimulating influences of air, light and water, elimination would become normal and general all over the body, and the complexion would soon clear up and become as pure and beautiful as that of a child. This we constantly prove in our work. Nature Cure is therefore the best and most rational of all cosmetics.

As explained in a previous chapter on density — dark discolourations, signs and spots stand for lack of blood, sluggish circulation, chronic catarrhal conditions and destruction of tissues in the corresponding parts and organs of the body; therefore the dark scurf rim is the sign of an enervated, vitiated skin, of poor surface circulation and of defective elimination. Anatomists have observed the scurf rim and attribute it to a weak, relaxed and shrivelled condition of the outer rim of the iris and to actual perforations of the surface layer, but they fail to give the causes of this abnormal condition. Figure 8 is copied from a standard work on anatomy. It shows the scurf rim (A), nerve rings (contraction grooves)(B), itch spots (C), sympathetic wreath (D) and chronic destructive lesions (E).

Pathogen and Skin Action

The question may be asked, how is it that persons without a scurf rim often suffer from defective skin action? In my explanations of pathogen obstruction in the capillary circulation I have brought out the fact that elimination through the skin may be diminished and checked by precipitation of uric acid or pathogen in the surface capillaries, the result of which in extreme cases would be complete cessation of elimination through the skin, and cessation of heat radiation. Weakening or suppression of the surface circulation by uric acid deposits in the capillaries (collaemia) may occur in people with otherwise good skin action as a result of faulty diet or disease of the kidneys. The degree of colloid or pathogen precipitation in the surface blood vessels may be accurately determined in the following manner by the reflux test: Press a finger tip on the skin. If the white patch thus produced fills up with blood immediately, say in three or four half-seconds, then the circulation is active and normal. If, however, the reflux of blood into the white patch occupies from four to twenty half-seconds, then the circulation is impeded by colloid or mucoid precipitates. The degree of occlusion can be estimated by the length of the time of the reflux.

How to Efface the Scurf Rim

Massing of the scurf rim in certain segments of the outer iris is always a sign of weakness and morbid incumbrance in the corresponding part of the body. If the scurf rim is very marked in the lower half of the iris and if the upper part, especially in the region of the brain, shows the whitish signs and clouds of inflammatory conditions, this is an indication that the circulation in the cutaneous surface and in the extremities is weak and sluggish and that as a consequence the inner blood pressure, especially in heart, lungs and brain is abnormally high (Fig.13). This may mean cold extremities, sluggish circulation in the portal system (stomach, bowels, liver and spleen), swollen veins on the legs, haemorrhoids, neuralgias, toothaches, colds, and catarrhs of the throat, lungs and nose, and high blood pressure or congestion in the heart, lungs and brain. From this it is apparent that in order to cure these various ills it is necessary to re-establish the normal activity of the skin, and this is best accomplished by the nude air baths, cold water baths, light, porous or no underwear, massage, neurotherapy and by a low protein diet free from pathogenic materials.

"But", I hear you say, "I cannot stand cold water. I might just as well die. Mr. So-in-So may stand it, but it would certainly kill me. Unless I wear the warmest clothing I freeze to death". Not so, Madam. Keeping warm is not a matter of piling on clothes, but of good skin action and reaction. We cannot make a weak arm strong by carrying it tied up in a sling. We must exercise it. We cannot make a weak, enervated skin strong and active by coddling it and by burying it under piles of dense, heavy underwear and clothes. People come to us in the summer wearing one or two thick suits of underwear, and then they are shivering and catching cold in every passing breath of air. A few weeks of cold water treatment, light, sun and air baths, massage and neurotherapy bring new life and blood into the surface, and the skin takes on the pink and rosy hue of life. Snakelike, these patients shed skin after skin of underwear, chest protectors, woollen stockings, gloves, overcoats, and the dead surface cuticle of their bodies, and then begin to enjoy contact with the life-giving elements. Like the Indian they can say "My body all face". The cuticle of their bodies has become as active, alive and immune to heat and cold as that of their faces. Many patients who come to us in such a weakened, sensitive condition are now taking regularly every day in the crisp January and February air, nude air baths. They do this not because we advise them to do so, for we refrain from prescribing such heroic treatment, but because they enjoy the sport.

Regeneration of the skin under a natural regimen is accompanied by a gradual decrease and often by a complete disappearance of the scurf rim. When the skin becomes active and alive, fine white lines become visible in the dark rim and these broaden out gradually into light patches. Since the scurf rim usually results from suppressive treatment and weakening, enervating influences which produce chronic conditions, it belongs as a sign in the iris to the third stage of encumbrance.

CHAPTER VIII

ITCH OR PSORA SPOTS
IN THE IRIS
(Fig.9, Colour plate, a and b)

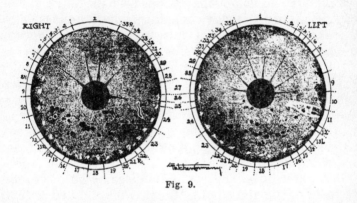

Fig. 9.

In civilised countries, especially in those bordering on the Mediterranean Sea, where suppression of itch and other skin eruptions is commonly practiced, about ten percent of all eyes show in the iris sharply defined dark brown spots ranging in size from that of a pinhead to that of a buckshot (Fig.8, also Fig.9 and Colour plate, a). These spots iridology designates as itch or psora spots, because they appear after the suppression of itchy eruptions or eczemata and of psoric parasites (pediculi capitis and pubis). I have observed in many instances that suppression of psoric eruptions resulted in formation or enlargement of the scurf rim instead of in the appearance of itch spots. This is probably due to the weakening of the skin by suppressive agents, such a mercurial or other poisonous salves, etc.

The word "psora" was adopted by Hahnemann, the
father of homoeopathy, from a Greek word signifying "itching", and he applied the name to certain skin diseases which
are characterized by intolerable itching. Probably no other
question in medical science has given rise to so much controversy as Hahnemann"s much disputed theory of psora. It is
therefore very interesting to observe in how far the eye confirms this theory of hereditary and chronic disease and in how
far it contradicts it.

The Theory of Psora

For one hundred years "Similia similibus curantur", the fundamental law of homoeopathy, has been the only fixed point
in the chaos of constantly changing medical theories, and in a
perverted form under the guise of vaccination, antitoxin,
serum and organ therapy, this great law of cure has been
adopted even by the allopathic school of medicine. Comparatively few of his closest friends and followers accepted
Hahnemann's theory of psora. This part of his teachings was
unmercifully ridiculed by his opponents and silently ignored
even by those who were believers in and exponents of the law
of "Similia". Briefly stated, the psoric theory claims that age
long persistent suppression of itchy, parasitic skin eruptions
and of gonorrhoeal and syphilitic diseases has encumbered
"civilised" humanity with three well defined taints or
miasms. These were named by Hahnemann psora or itch,
sycosis or gonorrhoea, and syphilis. He further claimed that
the greater part of chronic diseases had their origin in these
hereditary miasms and that many acute diseases are merely
external, palliative manifestations of these internal latent,
chronic taints.

Scurf Rim and Hereditary Psora.
(Fig.8a, 8c)

Darkening of the iris colour and the scurf rim stand for those
conditions which Hahnemann called "hereditary scrofula".
The name psora covers also those disease conditions which
result later in life from the suppression of itchy eczema,
hives, shingles, scabies (itch) and of other psoric parasites.
The itch or psora spots are never seen in the eyes of the new

born, but only later in life when psoric eruptions and
parasites have been suppressed by means of suplur, zinc or
mercurial ointments, by hot water, steam or hot air bathing,
or by any other agent or combination of methods. To recapitulate: Darkening of the iris colour and scurf rim stand for the
long list of hereditary ailments which Hahnemann calls
heredity psora, commonly known as "scrofulous diathesis".
The dark brown itch or psora spots and the scurf rim stand for
the effects of suppressed itch and psoric parasites. I have
observed that blue eyed parents suffering from suppressed
itch, as shown by the itch spots in the their eyes, usually have
brown eyed or "scurf rimmed" children. These revelations of
the iris confirm Hahnemann's statement that suppression of
acute itch or scabies creates hereditary psora and chronic
constitutional psora in the offspring.

Before we proceed in our study of the itch spots in the
eye it will be instructive and interesting to quote a few
passages from Hahnemann's "Chronic Diseases" and to learn
just what he means by psora and suppression of psora. Our
esteem and admiration of this wonderful man will be greatly
increased when we reflect that he discovered, by keenness of
intuition and by marvelous powers of concentration and
observation, what we today see so easily and plainly revealed
by iridiagnosis.

QUOTATIONS FROM HAHNEMANN"S
"CHRONIC DISEASES"

"Thus this eruption, externally reduced in cultivated countries to a common itch, could be much more easily removed
from the skin through various means, so that with the medical
external treatment since introduced, especially in the middle
and higher classes, through baths, washes and ointments of
sulphur and lead, and by preparations of copper, zinc and
mercury, the external manifestations of *Psora* on the skin
were often so quickly suppressed, and are so now, that in
most cases, either of children or of grown persons, the history
of itch infection may remain undiscovered.

"But the state of mankind was not improved thereby; in many respects it grew far worse. For, although in ancient times the eruption of Psora appearing as leprosy was very troublesome to those suffering from it, owing to the lancinating pains in and the violent itching all around the tumors and scabs, the rest of the body enjoyed a fair share of general health. This was owing to the obstinately persistent eruption on the skin, which served as a substitute for the internal Psora.

PSORA has thus become the *most infectious* and *most general* of all the chronic miasmas. For the miasm has usually been communicated to others before the one from whom it emanates has asked for or received any external repressive remedy against his itching eruption (lead-water, ointment of the white precipitate of mercury), and without confessing that he had an eruption of itch, often even without knowing it himself; yea, without even the physician's or surgeon's knowing the exact nature of the eruption, which has been repressed by the lotion of lead, etc...

"Mankind, therefore, is worse off from the change in the external form of the *Psora* — from leprosy down to the eruption of itch —not only because this is less visible and more secret and therefore more frequently infectious, but also especially because the *Psora*, now mitigated externally into a mere itch and on that account more generally spread, nevertheless still retains unchanged its original dreadful nature. Now, after being more easily repressed, the disease grows all the more unperceived within, and so, in the last three centuries, after the destruction of its chief symptom (the external skin eruption) it plays the sad role of causing innumerable secondary symptoms, i.e. it originates a legion of chronic diseases, the source of which physicians neither surmise nor unravel.

"So great a flood of numberless nervous troubles, painful ailments, spasms, ulcers (cancers), adventitious formations, dyscrasias, paralyses, consumptions and cripplings of soul, mind and body were never seen in ancient times when the *Psora* mostly confined itself to its dreadful cutaneous symptom, leprosy. Only during the last few centuries has mankind been flooded with these infirmities, owing to the causes just mentioned.

It was thus that PSORA became the *most universal* mother of chronic diseases.

1"It is incredible to what an extent modern physicians of the common school have sinned against the welfare of humanity, since, with scarcely an exception, teachers of medicine and the more prominent modern physicians and medical writers have laid down the rule and taught it as an infallible theorem that: "Every eruption of itch is merely a local ailment of the skin, in which ailment the remaining organism takes no part at all, so that it may and must be driven away from the skin at any time and without any scruple, through local applications of sulphur ointment or of the yet more active ointment of Jasser, through sulphur fumigations, but solutions of lead and zinc, but most quickly by the precipitates of mercury. If the eruption is once removed from the skin everything is well and the person is restored and the whole disease removed. Of course, if the eruption is neglected and allowed to spread upon the skin, then it may eventually turn out that the malignant matter may find opportunity to insinuate itself through the absorbent vessels into the mass of humours and thus corrupt the blood, the humours and the health. Then, indeed, man may finally be affliced with ailments from these maglignant humours, though these might soon again be removed from the body by purgatives and abluents; but through prompt removal of the eruption from the skin all sequelae are prevented and the internal body remains entirely healthy'.

"These horrible untruths have not only been, and are still being taught, but they are also being carried out in practice. The consequence is that at the present day the patients in all the most celebrated hospitals, even in those countries and cities that seem most enlightened, as well as the private itch patients of the lower and higher classes, the patients in all the

penitentiaries and orphan asylums, in other civil and military
hospitals, wherever such eruptions are found — in short, the
innumerable multitude of patients, without exception, are
treated, not only by physicians unknown to fame, but by all,
even those *most celebrated*, with the above mentioned external
remedies, using perhaps at the same time large does of
flowers of sulphur, and strong purgatives (to cleanse the
body, as they say). These physicians think that the more
quickly these eruptions are driven from the skin the better.
Then they dismiss the patients from their treatment as cured,
with brazen assurance and the declaration that everything is
now all right, without regarding or being willing to notice the
ailments which sooner or later are sure to follow; *i.e.* the *Psora*
which shows itself from within in a thousand different diseases. If the deceived wretches then sooner or later return
with the malady following *unavoidably* on such a treatment;
e.g. with swellings, obstinate pains in one part or another,
with hypochondriac or hysterical troubles, gout, consumption, tubercular phthisis, continual or spasmopdic asthma,
blindness, deafness, paralysis, caries of the bones, ulcers
(cancer), spasms, hemorrhages, diseases of the mind and
soul, etc., the physicians imagine that they have before them
something entirely new and treat it again and again according
to the old routine of their therapeutics in a useless and hurtful
manner, directing their medicines against phantom diseases;
i.e. against causes invented by them for the ailments as they
appear, until the patient, after many years" suffering continually aggravated, is at last freed from their hands by death,
the end of all earthly maladies".

Is the Itch Disease Local and of Purely
Parasitic Origin or is it Constitutional?

When the microscope revealed a minute, ugly looking
parasite as the apparent cause of itch eruptions, allopathy
jubilantly declared that Hahnemann's theory of psora was
thereby finally disposed of. The little mite which is blamed
for this disagreeable disease has been named by science, the
acarus scabies, or sarkoptes hominis. Under the microscope
the parasite presents a ferocious appearance, having a body
resembling that of a tortoise with the legs of a spider. His

body is studded with strong bristles by means of which he braces and supports himself in the flesh of his victims when burrowing his tunnels into the lower layers of the skin. It is the prick of these bristles in the flesh and the work of his voracious maw which causes the intolerable irritation peculiar to the disease . The insect is devoid of eyes and nervous system; it is all mouth, teeth and stomach. The male is the smaller and burrows in the surface layers of the skin, while the female is larger and digs its shafts deep down into the cutis vera, or true skin, where it taps and sucks the minute blood vessels. Orthodox science says:"Itch is never found without the acarus scabies, therefore the latter must be the disease". Since the discovery of bacteria allopathy has extended this local and parasitic conception of disease so as to embrace almost every known pathological condition. As a natural corollary of this theory, germ killing has become the basis of modern medical science.

Iridology, however, conclusively proves that Hahnemann after all was right and that allopathy is in error when it claims that the killing of the itch microbe and of the vermin which infest head and pubis, effectually terminates these diseases. For, after the killing of these parasites by means of sulphurous and mercurial ointments and other agents, sharply defined brown spots appear in certain parts of the iris and it has been conclusively proved that the areas in the iris displaying these psora spots correspond to the parts and organs of the body in which, after external suppression, the psoric poisons have concentrated. We are often asked, "How can you prove that the scurf rim or brown spots in the iris have any relation to suppression of skin eruptions, itch parasites and vermin?". Our answer to this is: "The diagnosis from the iris of the eye and the progress of chronic cases under natural methods of living and treatment conclusively prove these facts". Instances like the following come under our observation almost daily.

Clinical Proofs

A case of itch has been promptly cured with sulphur ointment and within a year there appears in the iris of this person, close to the pupil (area of the stomach), a sharply defined dark brown spot, and from that time on, the person is greatly troubled with chronic gastritis and later on with ulcers of the stomach.

A mother is horrified to find on the head of her little girl some lice. Within a few days the hair is full of nits and the vermin have increased to an alarming extent. The mother applies coal oil, or mercurial ointments, and the "nasty things" disappear from the surface — but not from the body, The psoric taints which nature was trying to eliminate, now reinforced by drug poisons and by the deadly miasms contained in the bodies of the parasites themselves, recede into the interior and in place of being distributed throughout the entire body they now concentrate in some vital part or organ, and chronic headaches, epilepsy, chorea, asthma, nervousness, sexual perversion, etc., are often the result.

Several years ago a lady belonging to a wealthy and refined family came to us for a diagnosis of her case. The left iris displayed in the region of the cerebellum a light brown spot, and I remarked, "You have suffered for many years with chronic headaches, nervousness, twitchings in the limbs and muscles, and with dizziness". All of this she confirmed and wanted to know the cause of her life-long suffering. "As a school girl", I continued, "you were troubled with head vermin and your mother treated them in the usual way". "Yes", she answered, "I remember distinctly, I was affected that way several times, but what has that to do with my ailments?". I explained to her that not external filth alone but internal uncleanliness as well, favours the development of these parasites; that like bacteria they subsist on constitutional poisons and act as nature's scavengers which purify the system of scrofulous and psoric miasms. I also informed her that in many instances natural treatment had reproduced the formerly suppressed conditions and warned her to avoid suppressive treatment if such a healing crisis should develop in her case. One day, after three months of natural treatment, she complained about intolerable itching of the scalp. A look into her eyes revealed that the brown psora spot was surrounded and interlaced by fine white lines, the signs of an approaching acute reaction. "You will have visitors very soon", I remarked. "What visitors do you mean, doctor?"

"The same kind that your mother killed some twenty-five years ago". Within a week after this conversation she entered my office and laughingly exclaimed, "Oh Doctor, not one visitor, but a million. I am just alive with them". "All right", I answered. "Be thankful they have come. This means a cure of your chronic ailments. Do not use anything now but a comb and cold water". "How lucky, Doctor, that you told me about this in advance. Without your warning I would surely have rushed to a drug store and have done the same thing over again". Her old friends remained with her for about two weeks and then disappeared as they had come. From that time on she was free from the "terrible periodical headaches" and nervous ailments which had troubled her since childhood. Possibly this psoric crisis prevented the development of insanity in later years. "Catching" in this case was absolutely out of the question, for she lived in the most refined surroundings and for three months cold water sprays and douches had been applied almost daily to head and body.

We are often asked the question: "Where do they come from — you do not believe that they come from the body itself?". We do not know, but we do know by frequent experience that when the body begins to eliminate scrofulous poisons we need not worry whence germs and microbes are to come. As carrion attracts vultures so the chronic miasms attract bacteria and parasites. Occurrences like the one related answer the oft repeated question, "Why stir up these disease miasms — why not leave them where they are, if their elimination causes so much trouble?". If allowed to remain their presence means much greater trouble in the future. Better a brief healing crisis than paresis, cancer or tuberculosis.

Cancer Grows in Psoric Soil

The psora spots in the eye solve to a large extent the mystery surrounding the nature and origin of malignant tumours and of tuberculosis. If we find a vital part or organ affected by suppressed itch we know that such a person is in great danger of developing cancer, sarcoma, tuberculosis or other malignant chronic diseases in the encumbered parts. With two exceptions so far in our practice, all cases of cancer we have cured have developed itchy, burning eruptions as healing crises. The two exceptions to the rule eliminated the psoric taints by means of furunculosis. The almost certain appearance of itchy eruptions as healing crises during the course of cancer is of great significance. It throws new light upon the true causes of this dreaded disease and positively confirms Hahnemann's theory of psora. Knowing these facts, is it wise to avoid an insignificant healing crisis and to run chances of developing cancer in later life, or is it better to give the organism a thorough house cleaning in order to eliminate the morbid miasms and thus preclude the possibility of malignant tumours and of other chronic destructive diseases? Medical statistics prove that during the last fifty years, among the common causes of death, cancer shows an increase of over 400 percent. This confirms our opinion that the more refined the old school of medicine becomes in the suppression of acute diseases and the more it contaminates the blood of our people with smallpox, serums, antitoxin and other disease products, the greater will be the increase in chronic destructive diseases.

The following is the history of another typical psora case and of its development under natural treatment: Mr B., of Chicago, had been a chronic invalid ever since childhood, "doctoring" continually for all sorts of ailments and growing worse instead of better. Four years ago he became so weak that he was obliged to give up his profession and the doctors declared his to be a hopeless case. An examination of his eyes by a practitioner of Natural Therapeutics showed a large itch spot in the region of the small intestine. The doctor, after a superficial glance into his eyes, suprised him with the remark: "Early in life you had the itch and it was suppressed. The poison then concentrated in the small intestine, causing chronic intestinal indigestion, irritation and occasional diarrhoeas. You are now in great danger of developing cancer in the affected parts". Mr B. at once admitted the correctness of the diagnosis. He stated that while the doctors had treated him for "stomach troubles" he had always felt and insisted that most of the difficulty was in the bowels. On closer inspection it was found that there were two separate and distinct itch spots, one overlying the other, indicating that the

itch must have been suppressed twice. Mr. B. corroborated
this also, saying that he remembered distinctly having been
twice "cured" of itch eruption with sulphur and mercurial
ointments. He was then informed that he could be cured
easily and thoroughly by strict adherence to pure food diet
and by systematic natural treatment, and that if the diagnosis
was correct itch eruptions would again manifest on the surface as healing crises. This, however, would not occur until
his system had been sufficiently purified and strengthened by
the natural regimen. Mr. B. much impressed by this accurate
diagnosis and prognosis of his case entered with enthusiasm
on the new plan of living and treatment. His improvement
from the beginning was remarkable. After the lapse of two
months, having passed through the first healing crises he
returned to work and for many years has not missed a day's
labour. A year afterward Mr B. reported remarkable improvement in every respect. Both patient and doctor, however,
were somewhat puzzled because so far there had been no
manifestation of itch skin eruptions and because the psora
spots in the iris had not changed or diminished to any considerable extent.

So far no homoeopathic remedies had been administered
and I prescribed psorinum, Hahnemann's great anti-psoric
remedy. The patient received one dose of psorinum C.M.
Nine days after this he broke out on arms and body with typical itch eruptions. At the same time he developed a violent
intestinal crisis manifesting as severe colic and diarrhoea.
One day he reported in alarm that his bowels were "passing
away" from him. On inspection it was found that these
"bowels" were the decayed casings of his diseased intestines.
This simultaneous external and internal crisis conclusively
proved the relationship between suppressed itch, itch spot in
the iris, chronic enteritis, itch eruption and internal crisis.
The itchy eruptions then disappeared and the bowels resumed
their normal activity. The treatment during this crisis consisted of fasting and the usual cold water applications, no
medicines of any kind being given. After this thorough house
cleaning the patient felt greatly improved in body and mind,
and an examination of the iris revealed the fact that the uppermost layer of the itch spot had disappeared, but the lower and

darker was still in evidence.

Six months afterward the patient, who had in the meantime continued in the right way of living and of treatment,
received another dose of psorinum, partly in order to stir up
the remaining psora and partly to prove whether or not the
first results had been merely accidental. Six days after he
received the remedy an acne-form eruption appeared on his
body. This lasted about three weeks and was accompanied by
a severe catarrhal condition of the nasal and respiratory
passages. This crisis also left him much improved in general
health. At the present date the remnant of the itch spot in the
iris is very small and has paled into a yellowish colour.

Homoeopathy a Branch of Natural Therapeutics

This remarkable case is instructive in many respects. It proves the correctness of the diagnosis from the iris of the eye,
the efficacy of natural diet and treatment, the truth of
Hahnemann's theory of Psora and of his law of "similia
similibus curantur". This is only one of many cases which
might be cited as positive proof of the laws and principles laid
down and demonstrated on these pages.

After reading this history of a psoric case our friend the
Homoeopath might be tempted to object — "Why bother with
other forms of natural treatment? After all, the homoeopathic
remedy had to do the work". No, I would reply, psorinum
alone did not do the work. It merely gave the final push and
pull to the psora encumbered cells, which aroused them into
acute activity. Natural treatment first had to purify and sen-
sitize the organism before the homoeopathic potency could
act. We use the "similia" together with our other natural
methods when indicated, but we find that in many cases
where the vitality is low and the organism heavily encumbered with disease and drug poisons, the remedy alone is too
weak to produce a reaction. When, however, the system has
been sufficiently purified of its grosser encumbrances and
when the entire body has been stimulated into vigorous activity, then a high potency of the similar remedy often accom-
plishes wonders. Natural Therapeutics means an harmonious
combination of all natural healing factors in accordance with
the fundamental laws of cure and with the individual charac-

terstics of the case. To treat serious chronic ailments with one
"pathy" or one method when many others are at our service is
too much like pulling a heavy load with one horse when
others are idle in the stable.

The following narrative is another remarkable verifica-
tion of Hahnemann's theory of psora and of the signs of psora
in the iris. About seven years ago four of our students, three
men and one woman, left our institution to assume positions
as nurses in a physical culture sanitarium. Each of them was
there infected by a patient suffering with itchy eruptions
(scabies). In spite of all natural treatment which that institution afforded, the eruptions persisted for several months.
Miss M., one of the nurses, wrote to me that she was suffering
terribly from the eruptions with no sign of healing and that the
others and herself had been given the alternative of submitting to mercurial treatment or leaving the institution. Two of
the men submitted to the mercurial treatment and suppression. The third, Mr. C., went into the country and allowed the
infection to run its course, aided by natural living, and nude
air baths and cold water treatment. When Miss M. came back
to us her appearance was such that she was obliged to seclude
herself from public view. Inside of two months she had fully
recovered and again took up her work as a nurse in our
institution.

The significant results of this remarkable crisis were as
follows: when she first came to us, three years before, she
was suffering from tuberculosis and in addition she had
almost lost her eyesight. The iris showed a very heavy scurf
rim, revealing a psoric or scrofulous constitution. Under
natural living and treatment she recovered sufficiently to take
up our institutional training, but when she left us the scurf rim
was still visible and quite heavy. After the itch crisis had run
its course the scurf rim entirely disappeared and since that
time she has enjoyed better health than ever before.

When Mr. C. first came to us he had several itch spots in
each eye. He suffered from many defects of a scrofulous constitution. This fact induced him to take up the study of
Natural Therapeutics. He also had improved greatly before
he left our institution but the itch spots were still visible in his
eyes. When I saw him soon after his return from life on the

farm, the itch spots had entirely disappeared from his iris. He has enjoyed perfect health ever since this remarkable healing crisis.

Mr. R., who had subjected himself to mercurial treatment, came to me about six months after the drug suppression of the scabies. An earlier examination of the iris had shown good density, a light scurf rim and no itch spots. On the occasion of his last visit almost one half of the iris was covered by a heavy black scurf rim. I do not know what has become of him since, but I am certain that his condition was not improved by the suppressive mercurial treatment.

I could relate hundreds of similar equally interesting cases of psoric encumbrances and elimination, but space does not permit.

Isopathy

Isopathy, the forerunner of homoeopathy by a few hundred years, was taught and practised by Paracelsus, the mystic philosopher and physician, and his disciples. Isopathy administers the products, that is, the morbid excretions, of a disease in order to cure the same disease. Instead of the "similar" it is the "same" as the disease, which is the meaning of isopathy. During an epidemic of cholera in the sixteenth century particles of faeces of the victims of the plague were given as medicinal remedies to cholera patients. Homoeopathy uses the isopathic remedies, such as psorinum, tuberculinum, siphilinum in highly triturated and potentized preparations. Allopathy (like the mediaeval quacks) administers the products of disease in the forms of serums, vaccines and antitoxins in crude, poisonous doses.

CHAPTER IX

COMPARISON OF FERMENTATION TO INFLAMMATION

There is a remarkable similarity between alcoholic fermentation and the processes of feverish and inflammatory diseases. Both are processes of oxidation or combustion, accompanied by increased activity and temperature. Both run a natural, orderly course and when properly managed bring about certain normal. beneficial results. When not controlled or when suddenly arrested and suppressed, both may result in permanently abnormal and undesirable conditions. Both processes depend on three essential factors:

Alcoholic Fermentation depends on —	Feverish and Inflammatory Diseases depend on —
(1) A watery solution Corresponding to	(1) Living blood and tissue
(2) Sugar Corresponding to	(2) Waste and morbid matter in the blood
(3) Yeast Corresponding to	(3) Microzymes, bacteria, viruses and parasites in blood and tissues.

The following may serve as an explanation of the preceding diagram. Modern allopathic materia medica is founded largely on the assumption that bacteria and parasites of their own accord create disease conditions. From this they draw the natural conclusion that to kill the germs is equivalent to curing the disease. Almost their entire therapeutic efforts are directed to discovering, killing and eliminating by poisonous drugs, serums, antitoxins and by the surgeon's knife, the bacteria and parasites of disease. The following demonstrations, however, will prove that the primary assumption of allopathy, as well as its resulting conclusions, are fallacious and that a practice built on these false foundations must of necessity be pregnant with disastrous results.

Comparison Between

Fermentation pure water	Inflammation pure blood and tissues
Yeast grows and multiplies in a sugar solution only; thrown into pure water it lies dormant and inactive.	Microzymes develop into bacteria and parasites only in pathogenic materials. They remain quiescent in a body possessed of pure blood and tissues and of normal vitality.

First or Hereditary Stage of Disease

Fermentation	Inflammation
Water plus a sugar solution (grape juice) Corresponds to	A body plus hereditary and acquired morbid matter

Second or Acute Inflammatory Stage of Disease

| Yeast lives on sugar plus some protein. While feeding on these, the yeast germ digests or splits up the sugar into alcohol and | Microzymes, while feeding on morbid matter, develop into bacteria or germs of putrefaction, and these in turn while feeding on |

carbonic acid gas.

Disintegration of the sugar molecules is accompanied by the liberation of heat and by accelerated atomic motion. The temperature rises perceptibly, bubbles of carbonic acid gas and a scum consisting of dead and live yeast germs and of other debris rise to the surface, Processes of fermentation are in many respects identical with processes of digestion, combustion or oxidation. The entire fermenting fluid is in violent commotion. If fermentation is allowed to run its natural course, within certain limitations of temperature, until all sugar in the fluid is consumed, the process ceases of its own accord. Chemical activity and temperature subside, and the resulting product is a wine-like fluid of crystal clearness. Alcohol, while itself the product of fermentation, as it accumulates in the fluid, checks fermentation.

pathogenic materials decompose them into simpler compounds suitable for neutralization and elimination. The resulting ashes or debris (see yeast scum) are eliminated through the natural channels of depuration and in the forms of pus, catarrhal and other morbid discharges. These processes of combustion and elimination of disease matter are usually termed fevers, inflammations, boils, abscesses, etc. Like fermentations they are accompanied by rise in temperature, accelerated (motion) pulse, elimination of effete matter, etc. If the acute inflammatory processes in the body are allowed to run their natural course, within certain limitations of temperature until all morbid matter is consumed and eliminated, the result is a cleaner, healthier body. (Fever can easily be controlled within safe limits by cold water applications, fasting, etc. The products of bacterial action tend to check bacterial growth and development.

From this it will be perceived that the processes of fermentation as well as of acute diseases are to a certain extent self-limited by their own effete products. If the acute activities in the body run their natural course and terminate in normal conditions, then the whitish signs of inflammation in the iris gradually disappear and give way to normal blue or brown. The second or acute stage of encumbrance as recorded in the iris of the eye is illustrated in Fig. 14, Series I, and Figs. 10-11.

Third or Chronic Stage of Disease

Fermentation

Inflammation

Yeast fermentation in a sugar solution may be promptly prevented or arrested by the addition of salicylic acid, formaldehyde or some other powerful antiseptic or germicide. Antiseptics are protoplasmic poisons, that is, they paralyze and destroy the protoplasm of living cells and inhibit their activity. Fermentation, suppressed by antiseptics, results in a turbid fluid containing unfermented sugar, dead yeast germs and poisonous antiseptics. Prof. Bechamp proved that yeast fermentation thus arrested by antiseptics results in decomposition of the yeast cells and the appearance of bacteria in their stead. These experiments were conducted

Acute inflammatory conditions in the body may be subdued or suppressed by protoplasmic poisons, such as antiseptics, antipyretics, opiates, sedatives, alteratives, or any other class of poisons which paralyze or destroy cell protoplasm and inhibit vital functions. All of these poisons not only paralyze and destroy bacteria and parasites of disease, but also paralyze and kill the healthy tissues of the body. If the acute, feverish and inflammatory reactions of the second stage of encumbrance are suppressed by antiseptics and germicides, the combustion and elimination of morbid matter is hindered and suppressed, and drug poisons, which are much more harmful than disease under conditions which made the invasion of bacteria from without an impossibility

poisons, are super-added to the old encumbrances of morbid matter.

These accumulations of effete and foreign matter become a source of continual irritation and obstruction, and form a luxuriant soil for the production or invasion of bacteria and parasites. In other words, nature's acute cleansing and healing efforts are changed into chronic catarrhal diseases.

The Chronic stage of encumbrance as recorded in the iris of the eye is illustrated in Fig.14, Series III.

Fourth or Chronic Destructive Stage of Disease
(Loss of Substance)

Fermentation

If the turbid fluid, created by the suppression of alcoholic fermentation, be exposed to air and warmth, its microzymes will develop into spurious germs and ferments and various forms of wild fermentation.

These spurious fermentations, in their turn, may be suppressed by more antiseptics and germicides, but as a result the fluid becomes totally unfit as a beverage and finally

Inflammation

The human organism, when it has reached the third stage of encumbrance, will arouse itself occasionally to feeble (chronic) efforts of elimination, but ever increasing accumulation of morbid matter, continual additions of drug poisons, surgical mutilations of vital parts and organs, all conspire to lower the vitality and to prevent the possibility of any decisive, acute reactions or healing poisonous to human life.

crises. The natural resistance and powers of reaction of the organism are in this manner slowly but surely undermined and weakened. Decay and destruction gradually proceed into the advanced stages of tuberculosis, malignant tumours, paralysis, agitans, locomotor atazia, paresis, pernicious anaemia, chronic rheumatism, etc.

These destructive changes of the fourth stage of encumbrance, as recorded in the iris of the eye are illustrated in Fig.14, Series IV.

The Making of a Chronic

In order to illustrate the foregoing theoretical expositions of the development of acute and chronic diseases by a living example from every day experience, I shall describe a typical case of consumption, tracing its various progressive stages to the fully developed tuberculosis, and thence to health under the regenerating influences of natural living and natural methods of cure.

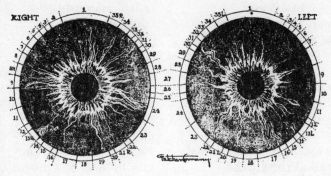

Fig. 10.

"John" was born with eyes of dark violet blue, indicating that "the sins of the fathers", that is, unnatural modes of living and of healing for many generations past, had endowed him with the undesirable inheritance of a psoric or scrofulous constitution. Nature, ever seeking to establish the perfect normal type, almost at birth began to eliminate the morbid inheritance through the skin and the mucous membrane of the digestive and respiratory tracts. (Fig.10). But these well meant cleansing and healing efforts of nature were misunderstood by John's parents and the family doctor. When the scalp took up the work of scrofulous elimination in the form of milk scurf and exzematous eruptions, it was smothered in oils, unsalted butter, cream, or mercurial ointments, in order to suppress as quickly as possible the "dreadful looking scabs". If the mother, after this "successful cure", had looked closely into the baby's eyes she would have noticed in the outer rim of the iris the appearance of a dark, broad ring — the "scurf rim" — and also a slight darkening of the iris colour in general (Fig.11). Mother Nature, however, does not give up the fight so easily. Thwarted in one quarter she tries in another. Liver, kidneys, stomach and bowels next took up the work of purification. Johnny had attacks of gastritis, vomiting, colic, and constipation alternating with diarrhoea. The scofulous poisons eliminating through the membranes of the intestinal tract bred worms of various descriptions. But the doctor, the grandmother, the aunt and the entire female neighbourhood within a radius of several miles, contributed advice, teas, drugs and salves of all possible descriptions to "cure" the pains, colics, worms, constipation and diarrhoea as fast as Mother Nature developed them. If the mother had examined Johnny's eyes as he passed through these periods of strenuous doctoring, she would have noticed around the pupil in the regions of the stomach and bowels the development of a peculiar wreath full of black spokes and spots, denoting the localities in stomach and intestines where drugs and suppressed disease poisons had accomplished their work of destruction (Fig.11). She would also have noticed various colour marks indicating the locations in which drug poisons had gradually accumulated. Fine, whitish nerve rings indicated that Johnny's nervous system, irritated and over stimulated by disease and drug poisons, was badly out of balance.

As the encumbrances of Johnny's system grew more serious and more complicated, nature's efforts at elimination became more drastic and severe. He was going to school now and his mother was very indignant because "he was catching from dirty children" every "infectious" disease within hailing distance. Now he would be down with the measles, then with scarlet fever, another time he was infected with lice and itch and, to cap it all, he was taken with smallpox. Mother and doctor failed to see that these "infectious" diseases were varied forms of psoric elimination. These "dreadful" diseases were also promptly "cured" by poisonous drugs and serums. That is, they were checked and suppressed before they had run their full and natural courses, and were thus made permanent in the form of defective hearing, liver and kidney diseases, indigestion and malnutrition (Figs.11-12). Though John, in his numerous trials with allopathic and home made remedies, did not contract and carry off all of the defects and blemishes mentioned above, he entered upon young manhood sufficiently handicapped to make life a burden. Suppression of psoric diseases left "itch spots" in his eyes in the regions of the liver, kidneys and intestines, indicating where the psoric poisons had concentrated (Figs.12-13). As a consequence, elimination through the natural channels was seriously impeded, but waste matter and poisons had to be disposed of somehow. The mucous membranes of throat, bronchi and lungs undertook this work of vicarious elimination for kidneys and bowels, and it is not to be wondered that John was "catching cold" with every passing draught.

Doctor Pills, who had "cured" so many of his childhood ills, now furnished the cheerful information that the catarrh and cough were becoming chronic. John continued to lose ground little by little. One day he walked into the doctor's office and remarked: "Well, Doctor, my feet got wet the other day and I caught another bad cold. I am coughing and expectorating terribly — it keeps me awake". "All right, John" answered the doctor, "here is some quinine sulph. that will down the fever; and here is some codein (opium) that will make you sleep and dry up that cough. Come back in a few days and let me see how you are getting on." After a few weeks John came again. "Well, Doctor, your medicine worked like a charm. The fever was gone in twenty-four hours and the coughing and spitting has almost stopped now. Only I feel so weak in my limbs and my back aches and I have such a depressing headache and then my bowels won't move at all." (Depressing effects of quinine and opium.) "All right, John, we'll fix that up for you. Here is some phenacetin that will stop your aches, and here is a nice tonic (arsenic, strychnine and iron) that will give you a fine appetite. And then you eat a good big beefsteak twice and day, eggs and chicken, soups and beef tea. A little beer or good old brandy won't hurt you either." "All right, Doctor, but what about the bowels?" "Oh yes, I forgot about them — here are some pills. Take a few after each meal. They will keep you going like clockwork." One month later; "Good morning, Doctor." "Good morning John, how are you?" "Well, Doctor, it might be better. That cough you stopped seems to be getting a little worse again, and I eat and eat, but I don't seem to grow any stronger — it feels like a big stone in my stomach. My bowels worked a little better for a while, but now they won't move at all. Then sometimes I have a bad pain in my chest, and I am growing quite short winded." "All right, John, I see we have to give it to you a little stronger. Here are some calomel pills (mercury) — take a few every night and follow it up in the morning with a good dose of salts. This is bound to do the work. Your appetite will be better, you will eat more and that will give you more strength. I notice your heart and pulse are getting a little weak. I'll give you some digitalis; that will strengthen your heart. And here is some ipecac to loosen the mucous in your lungs and help to bring it up."

Another month went by and poor John was not quite well yet. Once in a while he had a time of feeling well, and then the doctor told him the medicine was doing splendidly; again John was worse, and the doctor said he must give him something stronger. By and by John became impatient. He thought "all that medicine" should have benefited him in some way. He did not like to leave his doctor, since Dr. P. now "knew his system" so well. He imagined that if he went to another doctor now, the latter would have to "study his system" for a year or so before understanding his multitudinous ailments. Dr. P.

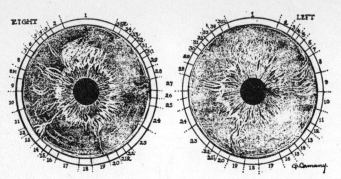

Fig. 11.

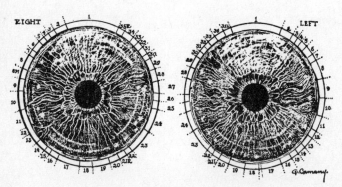

Fig. 12.

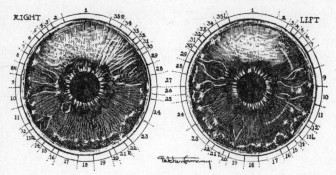

Fig. 13.

himself grew somewhat tired of the case. It grated on his nerves to see poor John come again and again with the same old "tale of woe". He knew that the patient could not last much longer and advised him to see a celebrated lung and throat specialist. John's vitality had been more and more lowered by the long continued effects of stimulants and virulent poisons. Poisonous tonics had worn out his stomach and cathartics his bowels. Quinine, iodine, arsenic, etc., were racking his flesh and bones with neuralgic pains. Degeneration of the lungs had progressed far enough to form a luxuriant soil for the tubercle bacilli. The celebrated lung specialist examined the sputum and found the bacilli in great numbers. He then proceeded to kill the germs with coal tar products (Fig.13). But these poisons did not stop to pick out just the bacilli. On their way through the body they also destroyed red blood corpuscles and delicate tissues of vital organs. So, between the germs and the germ killers, the tonics and the over feeding, the mercury, salts and other good old orthodox pills and potions, John in spite of all that money and science could do for him, went rapidly from bad to worse.

The Resurrection

Finally the great lung specialist, recognizing the futility of his efforts, ordered John to pack his trunk as quickly as possible for El Paso or Phoenix, the paradise of "one lungers". Finding himself (thanks to long continued illness and expensive doctoring) short of the necessary funds required for an extended sojourn in the southern mecca of consumptives, John decided as a last and forlorn hope to obtain my opinion of his case.

Evidently having been informed about our way of doing things, he asked me to examine his eyes and give him a correct inventory and an estimate of his remaining anatomy. While I found some parts missing and others badly damaged, I did not consider his case entirely hopeless. From the records in the iris I proceeded to unravel his history as outlined in the preceding sketch. When the diagnosis was finished he asked me whether I "got it" psychometrically or mediumistically. I assured him that I did not have to draw on any supernatural powers; that, on the contrary, my "reading" from the iris was

based on very simple and strictly scientific facts and principles. By means of a magnifying mirror and a chart of the iris
he was himself able to locate and to recognize the principal
landmarks. He had to admit that the record in his eyes exactly
tallied with his past history and present symptoms, and he felt
convinced that there was "something in it". I assured him that
though his case was somewhat complicated and advanced, I
by no means considered him incurable since he possessed
youth, some hundred and thirty pounds of flesh and the odds
and ends of an originally good constitution. Only an actual
trial could determine the possibility of cure. If there was left
in his organism sufficient vitality and if his kidneys were not
damaged beyond repair, his system would soon respond to the
purifying and invigorating influences of natural treatment.

Furthermore, it was explained to him that when properly
assisted nature always works her cures in a perfectly orderly
manner, in harmony with certain well defined laws of crisis
and periodicity. In conformity with these laws there would be
about six weeks of general improvement especially noticeable in the digestive organs. First of all the bowels, which, in
spite of laxatives and cathartics, had been sluggish and constipated for a lifetime, would begin to act normally and freely.
Then, as his system became purified and invigorated, nature
would commence in earnest her work of elimination and
repair. Febrile diseases and skin eruptions long ago suppressed, as shown in the iris, would reappear and this time
run their course in regular, natural order. I also informed him
that during these crisis periods he would experience various
symptoms of acute poisoning such as are commonly produced by quinine, coal tar products, mercury, iodine, etc.,
because these drug poisons accumulated in the course of
many years would be stirred up in their lairs and would be
eliminated in due season each under its peculiar symptoms.
When I had proceeded thus far in my prognosis John arose
somewhat abruptly, grabbed his hat and started for the door,
saying he would come back some other time — that he must
now hasten to keep another important appointment. Reading
his thoughts, I assured him there was no cause for alarm; that
the healing crises come in mild form only, because they cannot materialize until the system is properly prepared, and in a

healing crisis nature always has the best of the fight. I also called his attention to the fact that he was rapidly wasting away in destructive disease crises and unless a speedy change was wrought in his condition he would soon be beyond the possibility of healing crises. Reassured and encouraged by my explanation he decided to give Natural Therapeutics a fair trial.

I then proceeded to inquire into his daily habits and to offer suggestions for their correction. He was instructed that if he wished to eliminate old accumulations of disease and drug poisons he must stop taking in new ones in the form of meat, alcohol, drugs, coffee or tea. The patient was put on a vegetarian, but withal positive, diet; everything in impure food and harmful drinks was promptly eliminated from his diet. This greatly relieved his organs of elimination and gave them a chance to remove old encumbrances of morbid matter and poisons. Cold water treatments, massage, spinal manipulation, simple health gymnastics, normal suggestion and the indicated homoeopathic remedies, all contributed to increase in a natural and harmless manner the activity of skin, bowels, kidneys, mucous membranes and in fact of every cell in the body, and this increase of activity was brought about without introducing into his system any poisons whatsoever. No condition can be called incurable until a combination of all these natural healing factors has been tried and has failed. If there be vitality enough to react properly under such treatment and if the destruction of vital parts be not too great the system will soon respond. John's case, fortunately, was of this description. Under our treatment the worst symptoms of the patient rapidly abated, his appetite improved wonderfully, the bowels moved more freely than for many years past; he grew in strength physically and mentally. He continued thus to improve for about two months, all the while watching with us for the predicted manifestations. Then he came to us and said: "I do not believe your crises are going to materialize in my case — I suppose I was not sick enough to have any. Don't you think I might go home now?" I smilingly answered: "Just wait a bit and see — you will whistle a different tune by and by."

A few days later our erstwhile too confident patient

came to see me in a different frame of mind — the picture of
fright and despair. "Oh my, Doctor, I must have caught a terrible cold, but I cannot imagine where, unless it was that last
cold water treatment. I told the attendant he was putting it on
too long and too cold, but he only laughed at me, — and now
I've got it. And those nuts I ate did not agree with me, either —
I am always a little afraid of them. I'm just as constipated and
nauseated as I was six weeks ago. I have chills and fever and
the cough and catarrh are worse than ever. I feel it is all up
with me now. It's too bad, after having been so hopeful and
confident of recovery. I suppose I was too far gone and my
friend Jack was right. He told me this kind of cure was all
right for rheumatism, but starvation diet and cold water
would surely kill me." Without wasting any sympathy on him
I congratulated him on his good fortune, jokingly saying —
"Well, well, such a beautiful crisis. And just on time too. Oh,
these crises. They are so pleasant to talk and read about and
they are really interesting when it's on the other fellow, but
when they strike us we wish the doctor and his Natural
Therapeutics in a warmer clime and feel like making a short
cut for the drug store 'to have something done quickly'. Oh,
yes, you thought you were not going to have any crisis; well,
without doubt it has you now. No, you will not die; don't
worry — you are doing gloriously. If you don't feel like eating, fast until you are hungry. If you feel hot and feverish,
take a cold sponge or a foot bath; or if you have the chills and
cannot get warm, take a wet pack and a hot drink. This
together with our regular treatment will be fully sufficient for
any emergency, and nature will do the rest." My good humour
and confidence, inspired by absolute knowledge of the law,
were more effective than the pills and blisters of Dr. P. John
had it out with his fever, coughed, expectorated, perspired
and had a pretty tough time of it generally. Notwithstanding
the seeming severity of the symptoms he was able to attend to
his usual duties with remarkable ease and endurance. Nature
had the best of it — she never undertakes a healing crisis
unless the organism is in a condition to conduct it to a successful termination.

After a few weeks of crisis our patient began to improve
growing stronger day by day. He realized he had actually

"gotten rid of something" — he felt remakably light and energetic, in fact better than for many years. I warned him, however, not to be over elated and not to mistake the first period of real improvement for a permanent cure. For, while the eyes showed greatly improved conditions in lungs, bronchi and digestive organs, they still revealed plenty of work ahead for nature's healing forces. And subsequent events again confirmed the records in the iris. After periods of "building up" and of splendid improvement, there would suddenly develop an inflammation of the kidneys, a 'bilious spell", symptoms of acute quinine, iodine or mercurial poisoning. But the climax was capped by an acute attack of pneumonia. His friends expected this to be the beginning of the end, but the inflammation in the lungs ran its course in less than two weeks and the patient began to improve, at first slowly and then more rapidly. Today, three years after the great crisis, he is in good health and enjoying life in Europe.

The Moral of It.

What lessons are to be learned from this remarkable and authentic case? The diagnostic signs in the eyes of this patient were verified — (1) by his previous history; (2) by his "symptoms" which exactly corresponded with the signs in the iris; (3) by his subsequent healing crises; (4) by the gradual disappearance of the signs and colour marks in the iris after the occurrence of healing and cleansing crises. The diagnosis from the iris as illustrated and confirmed by this and other cases, absolutely and conclusively proves the cumulative effect of drug poisons in the body. It demonstrates that everything which is foreign, uncongenial or injurious to life reveals its presence in the body by certain well defined colour marks in the iris of the eye. It furthermore proves conclusively that certain elements which in the organic form are normally present in the human organism, will become abnormal and injurious to health when taken in large doses in the inorganic mineral form. For instance, iron, sulphur, sodium, lime, phosphorus, magnesium and manganese, in the live organic form in fruits and vegetables may be taken continuously in large amounts without "showing" in the iris. The same elements, however, when taken in much smaller quan-

tities in the inorganic form, soon accumulate in those parts of
the body for which they exhibit a special affinity. These
accumulations of foreign matter reveal their presence and
location by well defined colour marks in the corresponding
areas in the iris of the eye.

Why is inorganic matter so injurious to living organisms?
Nature never intended coarse inorganic minerals to serve as
foods and medicines for human bodies. Evolution consists in
ever accelerated vibratory activity, accompanied by an
increasing refinement of matter and by greater complexity of
structure. In accordance with this law of evolutionary
development, each lower kingdom refines and prepares food
materials of the soil into the living protoplasm of the vegetable cell and thus prepares them for animal and human food.
The animal life principle refines and elaborates vegetable
matter into the highly refined and complicated molecular
structures of the animal cell. The vegetable lives on the
mineral, and the animal on the vegetable. To introduce the
coarse, inorganic forms of the mineral kingdom into the
animal organism is contrary to nature's plan. This explains
why nature did not prepare animal and human organs of
assimilation and elimination to cope with coarse, heavy
aggregations of the mineral kingdom; why animal and human
organisms cannot mould these uncongenial elements into
normal living tissues; and why the organs of depuration cannot eliminate them completely. As a consequence, such
foreign materials accumulate in parts of the organism for
which they possess a special affinity, and even afterwards,
unless eliminated by powerful, natural methods of treatment,
act as irritants and poisons, thus causing a large percentage of
chronic diseases.

What does diagnosis from the iris teach with regard to
the dogmas of Christian Science? If there is no disease, why
does God, or Nature, with marvellous exactitude, portray in
the iris of the eye every passing or permanent condition which
we are in the habit of calling disease? "Scientists" claim that
diseases are only "errors of mortal mind". Mortal mind,
however, until a few years ago never suspected the existence
of these records in the eyes. How then could it be instrumen-
tal in producing them? If the teachings of Christian Science be

true, we must necessarily conclude that the great Universal Intelligence which creates these wonderful records in the eyes is afflicted with a badly "erring mortal mind".

About a year ago I attended a gentleman, who, in addition to natural treatment, desired also the assistance of a Christian healer. One day at the bedside of our mutual patient I met the healer, a grand old man with the venerable head and features of a patriarch. In the course of our conversation he related to me the circumstances of his conversion and development as a faith healer. Twenty years before, while living in a small Texas town, he was stricken with typhoid fever. The local country doctors fed him as usual on calomel (mercury), quinine and salts. But in spite of their faithful services he did not improve and they finally pronounced his inevitable doom. In his last extremity he had recourse to the Bible. The promises and assurances of spiritual healing therein aroused new hope and confidence, he "threw physic to the dogs" and put his sole and entire reliance in the healing power of the Spirit. A powerful therapeutic faith, thus aroused, greatly invigorated and harmonized his mental vibrations and these in turn, by continuity, acted as a powerful tonic on the waning forces of the physical organism. Unhindered by poisonous drugs and stimulated by therapeutic faith, nature's healing forces now gained the ascendancy and the disease crisis was transformed into a healing crisis. But, he, as he assured me, attributed his marvellous recovery to a special intervention of the Lord. Through twenty years he had undoubtedly done a great deal of good in fighting the darkness and despair of crass materialism by a living faith in a higher spiritual healing power. But through all these years he had failed to understand the modus operandi of this healing power of nature and could not appreciate its limitations. Looking into his big blue eyes I saw the yellow colour marks of chronic quinine poisoning and as a concomitant the signs of chronic catarrh in the regions of the head, bronchi and lungs. After he finished his story I asked him the question: "Is it not a fact that you suffer from time to time with ringing in the ears, frontal headaches and nasal and bronchial catarrh?" To which he answered: "Yes, brother, that is true; though prayer has helped me these twenty years in every other ailment, the Lord has never cured me of this chronic catarrh."

Confessions like these I hear continuously from the lips of healers and Scientists. If Brother C. had understood the laws of cure as explained in these writings, he would have seen nothing remarkable in his spontaneous recovery from typhoid or from any other acute ailment, because they are in themselves healing and cleansing efforts of nature. He would also have understood that even the Lord could not cure him of his chronic catarrh so long as quinine, the primary cause and excitant of it, was not removed from his system; he would have known that it takes more than the buoyant and stimulating effect of therapeutic faith to eliminate such poisons from the system. With all due respect for the holiness and effectiveness of prayer, it is still true that a four months' thorough course of water cure, manipulative, dietetic and homoeopathic treatment would have accomplished a great deal more in diminishing the signs in the iris and the catarrh in the body than his twenty years of faithful prayer. After all, God helps those who help themselves, and the grandest and most efficient of all prayers is intelligent, well directed work.

CHAPTER X

EDITOR'S FOREWORD

In this and subsequent chapters Lindlahr deals with the signs in the iris of the various inorganic minerals which find their way into the body either by accident or by being used in medication of the allopathic kind, There is no doubt that in certain respects the information given in these chapters must be regarded as incomplete and out of date. There have been many changes in the practices of orthodox medicine since Lindlahr's time. For instance, the use of mercury in medication has very much declined and it may be said that in general the administration of drugs and their preparation have become much more subtle and less crude than they were half a century ago. Also antibiotics have to a great extent taken the place of drugs in the treatment of conditions which are believed to be due to infections by bacteria or viruses.

SIGNS OF INORGANIC MINERALS IN THE IRIS OF THE EYE

We are frequently asked, "Why do you presume to say what is natural to the system — how do you judge what is poisonous?" Nature answers these much disputed questions, as she does so many others, in the iris of the eye. Substances congenial to the body, those in which in quality and quantity normally belong to it, do not show in the iris. But all substances foreign or poisonous to the organism may reveal their presence and location by certain well defined signs and discolourations in the corresponding areas or fields of the iris. For hundreds of years physicians and scientists have disputed as to the advisability of introducing into the human body in foods and medicines, mineral and earthy elements in the inorganic mineral form. Homoeopaths, eclectics and physio-medical physicians seceded from the allopathic school of medicine because they condemned the use of inorganic materials in so-called physiological doses as medicines. Nature Cure advocates, from the very beginning of the movement, strongly empahsized the fact that even those minerals and earthy elements which naturally belong to the human body must be taken as food only in the live, organic form in vegetable or animal protoplasm. They claimed that iron, lime, sodium, potassium, magnesium, sulphur and phosphorus, though they are of the greatest importance in the vital economy of the body, must not be taken in the inorganic,

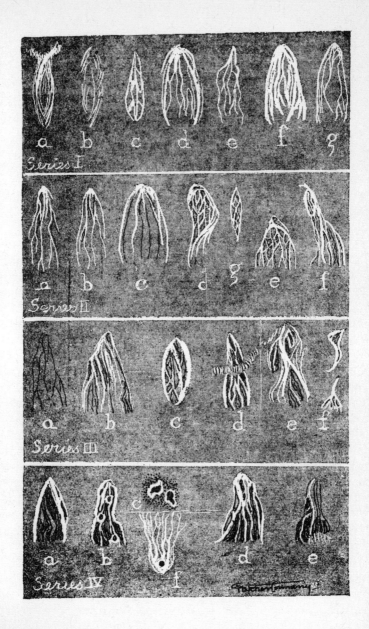

mineral form, lest they accumulate and concentrate in certain parts or organs of the body for which they exhibit a special affinity and there become harmful and dangerous to health and life. The student should carefully study Vol.1, Chap. XXIV, in which this subject is fully treated.

Previous to the discovery of nature's records in the iris, the question as to whether inorganic elements are beneficial or harmful to the human organism was largely a matter of opinion and controversy. No positive proof in support of either position was available. Iridology now proves beyond the shadow of a doubt that these substances, when taken in the inorganic form, accumulate in certain parts or organs for which they have a special affinity, as shown in our colour plate.

Colour Plate

Before beginning the description of the various colour signs in the iris I must call attention to the fact that the iris of perfectly normal human beings exhibits only one of two normal colours — a light azure blue for all pure blooded descendants of the Celtic and Indo-Caucasian races, and a pure light brown for the first three Aryan subraces and for the descendants of the fourth or Atlantean root race. From this it follows that any other colour pigments or discolourations of the iris indicate either abnormalities, disease processes or the presence of foreign matter or poisons in the system. The Iridologist, therefore, carefully studies every colour pigment in the iris and endeavours to discover its significance. While in this way a great deal of positive knowledge has been acquired concerning disease processes and the presence and exact location of foreign and toxic materials in the system, much remains to be explained in this intensely interesting field of scientific research. The effects upon the system of the various poisons exhibited in the iris are described elsewhere in this volume under the respective drug headings. The irides on this colour plate represent right eyes only. It is interesting to note that the pigments in the iris closely resemble the natural colour of the corresponding drugs.

Description

Fig.a — Blue eye.   This is a typical drug eye. The dark blue underground is covered with a whitish film produced by coal tar poisons, such as salicylic acid and creosote, and other poisons. The crescent in the upper margin of the iris is arcus senilis or gerontoxon. In the medical works it is described as an opacity of the upper margin of the iris. It is usually observed in people of advanced age, therefore the name. It is supposed to be a sign of lowered vitality and resistance of the organism as a whole and the brain tissues in particular. We frequently notice similar encroachments of the cornea on other sections of the iris. They are indicative of a weak lymphatic condition of the tissues and of low vitality. The arcus senilis must not be mistaken for certain drug signs which are described in this volume.

The inner margin of the arcus shows a yellowish discolouration caused by some drug poison, probably quinine. In the upper half of the iris, in the brain region, is displayed a broad crescent, the sign of potassium bromate and of other bromine combinations. The colour of the crescent varies according to the various chemicals associated with bromine in medical prescriptions. Sometimes the crescent covers the upper border of the iris and is extended more or less around the outer margin. It then shows similarly to the sodium ring in the same iris picture.

The broad whitish deposit all around the outer margin of the iris was caused by the absorption of large quantities of sodium bicarbonate (common baking soda). A similar deposit is formed by various substances containing large amounts of sodium, such as sodium salicylate, sodium sulphate, sodium bromate, etc. The salts of lime, magnesium and potassium show in similar manner. The location of the "salt ring" indicates that these mineral elements tend to concentrate and locate in the outer muscular structures of the body and in the skin, also in the brain tissue where they may have a serious effect upon memory and mental processes.

The white wheel in the stomach region, directly around the pupil, indicates the presence of strychnine in this organ. The sign is easily recognized by its perfect circular outline resembling a wheel and the uniform structure of its tiny spokes. The strychnine wheel appears imperfectly in Fig.f, where it is overshadowed by the sign of atrophy of the digestion organs.

The area of the intestinal tract surrounding the strychnine sign shows the rust brown discolouration of iron. In many instances this characteristic iron rust pigment covers the entire gastro-intestinal area. Inorganic iron has an astringent, benumbing effect upon the tissues. Its sign therefore indicates a sluggish, atrophic condition of the digestive organs. We frequently observe the sign in the eyes of people who have long used drinking water heavily charged with iron.

The sharply defined brown spots in the lower half of the iris are itch or psora spots. They are the signs of suppressed scabies or other itchy skin eruptions or eczemata as described in Chapter VIII. As time elapses after the suppression of psoric eruptions the itch spots grow darker in colour until they become blackish brown.

Fig.b — Blue eye.   The bright red spots in the iris are the sign of iodine. We find them in a large percentage of human eyes (in civilized countries). They are of a brighter shade of red or brown than the psora spots, and their outlines are more diffuse.

The whitish "snowflakes", mostly visible in the lower half of the iris, are the signs of arsenical poisoning. Their presence in the spleen, as in this case, often signifies enlargement of the spleen and the serious symptoms which go with it. The white flakes of arsenic are easily distinguished from the lymphatic rosary in the outer margin of the iris, visible in the form of white flakes on the inner border of a portion of the scurf rim. The lymphatic or typhoid rosary is more plainly visible in Figures c and e.

The scurf rim is the dark deposit on the outer margin of the iris, it being covered in the upper part by the white deposit. Where it extends all round the iris, as in this case, it dates back to infancy and indicates congenital scrofula or psora. If it appears only in parts of the iris, in crescent form, it has been acquired later in life.

The white deposit in the upper half of the iris, particularly the brain region, indicates the destructive effect of

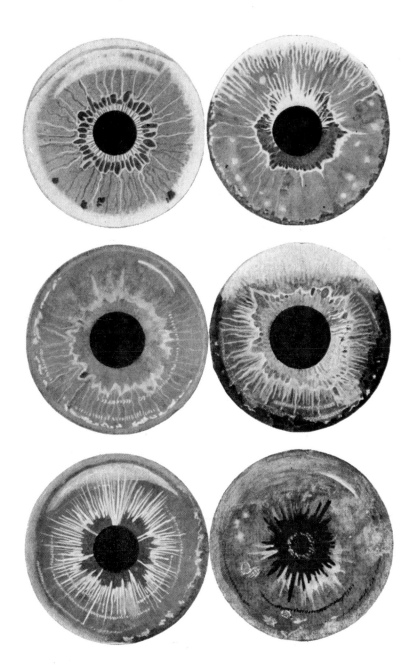

mercury and coal tar poisons upon the brain tissues, aggravated by bromides and the salts of other metals. We observe such bad demarcation and frazzled appearance of the upper rim of the iris frequently in the eyes of people threatened with or affected by apoplexy, insanity or paresis.

The purple discolouration in the area of the digestive organs indicates lead poisoning. We frequently find this in the eyes of printers, painters and others who work with lead. The white rays extending from the upper margin of the pupil to the brain region are the sign of opium, cocaine or morphine poisoning. In the eyes of drug fiends the white rays extend from all round the iris, partly from the pupil and partly from the sympathetic wreath.

The heavy, white sympathetic wreath surrounding the digestive area shows the effects of opiates and of powerful coal tar poisons, such as phenacetin and antipyrin, upon the sympathetic nervous system. In similar manner the sympathetic wreath may show the peculiar colour pigments of other poisons, such as the yellow colour of quinine, or reddish colour of iodine.

Fig.c — Blue eye.   This iris shows plainly the yellowish discolouration of quinine in the upper part of the iris, in the brain region, on the sympathetic wreath and in the region of the liver. The imposition of the yellow on the blue of the iris produces a greenish tint. This makes the "green" eye. While quinine has a special affinity for the brain and sympathetic system, we find its sign also in the areas of stomach, bowels, liver and spleen in the eyes of people who have taken considerable quantities of the drug for the treatment of malarial fevers, colds, hay fever and other forms of acute and chronic catarrh.

The outer rim of the iris shows the greenish ring of mercury. We found it difficult to reproduce this plainly. It requires some practice to distinguish it in the living eye. The small white crescent in the upper right margin of the iris indicates gummata — "softening of the brain" — the result of the destructive action of the mercury on the brain tissues. Those who plainly exhibit this sign usually suffer from some form of paralysis and are approaching the end of their suffering.

The lymphatic or typhoid rosary shows plainly in parts

of the outer margin of the iris. The fields of diaphragm and
sexual organs exhibit the brownish signs of ergot, in this case
administered for haemorrhage in childbirth. The triangle of
the pancreas contains a psora spot. The person who exhibited
this sign was in the last stages of diabetes.

An iodine spot shows in the lower back. It is partly surrounded by white indicating that the poison is in the process
of elimination. The patient who exhibited the sign told us that
during the eliminating crises he distinctly noted the iodine
taste. Elimination took place largely through furuncles.

The lower part of the iris exhibits plainly several sections of white nerve rings.

Fig.d — Brown eye.   The greyish wash over the upper
part of the iris indicates antikamnia poisoning. This is one of
the coal tar products commonly used for the treatment of
headaches, neuralgia and neuritis of the head. Iridiagnosis
plainly reveals the fact that the poison has a special affinity
for the brain region, more so than other coal tar products. We
have traced many cases of insanity to the effects of this drug
on the brain.

The yellowish discolouration in the region of the
stomach and bowels may be caused by sulphur or by
scrofulous elimination after the suppression of skin eruptions
in childhood. It must not be confounded with the yellow
colour of quinine which appears only in spots and clouds.

The sympathetic wreath with its white rays shows somewhat similarly to that of Fig.b; the explanation is the same.

The scurf rim is very broad and dark, indicating suppression of exzematous skin eruptions by metallic poisons.

The grey cloud in the region of the kidney, bladder and
genital organs is caused by turpentine. This substance has a
special affinity for the kidneys. The nerve rings in this iris are
turning dark indicating that nervous irritation is becoming
chronic.

The lymphatic rosary is visible in places through the
heavy scurf rim.

Fig.e — Brown eye.   About two-thirds of the outer
margin of the iris exhibits a heavy salt ring; the inner one-
third is covered by an "acquired" scurf rim.

The nerve rings show white, indicating acute nervous

irritation. The lymphatic rosary shows on the inner margin of the scurf rim. The large crescent in the brain region indicates deposits of bromides and other metallic salts.

The black discolouration in the digestive area stands for a sluggish, atrophic condition of the membraneous linings of stomach and bowels, produced most probably by the use of opiates and powerful cathartics from early youth in the form of paregoric, calomel, etc.

Fig.f — Brown eye.   This is a typical mercurial eye. The bluish rim in a brown eye indicates the presence of the poison in the system and its destructive effect upon the cuticle. The patient received many inunctions of mercurial ointments. The destructive effect of the poison on the brain tissues is revealed by the white crescent near the right upper margin of the iris.

The upper portion of the iris is covered with the greyish wash of coal tar products. The paralyzing effect of mercury and other poisons on the digestive tract is revealed by the black colour in the corresponding area. Only the inner margin of the stomach region shows faintly the strychnine wheel. Much strychnine was given to overcome the paralyzing effect of mercury and other drug poisons.

The white rays emanating from the digestive area indicates opiates taken to deaden the pain of locomotor ataxia. The red spots edged with white are typical of potassium iodide. We frequently find them in the spinal area of mercurial patients. This patient being in the last stages of mercurial destruction, commonly called tertiary syphilis, the nerve rings show black, indicating the atrophic condition of the nervous system.

Greyish clouds in the region of the throat and in the lower margin show the presence of glycerin. The yellowish flakes in the lung region are caused by phosphorus which was administered in the form of nerve stimulants.

The Sign of Iron (Fe) Ferrum
(Colour Plate, Fig.a.)
We find that iron, after it has been taken in considerable quantities in the inorganic form, shows in the areas of stomach and bowels as a rust brown discolouration which

closely resembles the colour of iron rust (Colour plate, a). I
have verified this sign in hundreds of cases in people who had
absorbed iron in inorganic form in medicines or in water
strongly impregnated with the mineral. Cases like the following have been of frequent occurrence: Several years ago a
lady came to one of our public clinics for a diagnosis from the
iris. The area around the pupil corresponding to the region of
the stomach and intestines, showed a very heavy iron discolouration. I asked whether she had not taken the mineral in
some form of drugs or patent medicines, but this she
positively denied. Adroit quizzing finally brought out the fact
that for several years she had used water from the iron spring
in Lincoln Park. After forming this habit she had suffered
much from constipation and indigestion. I explained to her
that these ailments were probably the result of the iron
poisoning. Following my advice, she adopted a pure food
natural diet and began a course of eliminative natural treatment. Within six months the iron sign had disappeared from
her eyes and the digestive organs were in normal condition.

Iron
Allopathic Uses:
   1. Externally on mucous membrances and broken skin as
constringent and striptic against diffuse haemorrhages,
catarrhal discharges and other inflamatory exudates.
   2. Internally the non-astringent preparations are used as
haematinics together with such drugs as influence the diseased conditions on which the anaemia or debility depend, for
instance:
   3. Iron arsenate in chronic skin affections, particularly
lupus, lepra, psoriasis, eczema, scrofula and syphilitic
lesions.
   4. Iron sulphate in chronic diarrhoea, dysentry and
passive haemorrhages accompanied by marked relaxation.
   5. Iron bromide or iodide as tonic-alterative in atonic
amenorrhoea and chlorosis in young women.
   6. Iron glycerophosphate and iron manganese during
convalescence, asthenic nervous conditions and rickets.
   7. Iron valerianate, in hysterical complaints complicated
with chlorosis.

8. Iron and quinine in malarial cachexia, cardiac disease and nephritis.

9. Antidote in acute arsenical poisoning, repeatedly administered in form of dialysed iron.

Accidental Poisoning:

1. Mineral waters.
2. Proprietary blood tonics.

Toxicology:

1. Unabsorbed and excreted as iron sulphide, colouring stools black.
2. Dyspepsia. Stubborn constipation.
3. Abdominal pain relieved by pressure.

Sodium (Na) Natrium

Sodium shows in the eyes in the form of a white wreath in the outer margin of the iris (See Colour plate, Figs. a and e). Before I became acquainted with Nature Cure, my eyes were heavily marked with drug signs. Some of these have entirely disappeared. Others are still faintly visible. Fig.15 is a reproduction of charts of my eyes drawn fourteen years ago by Dr. Henry Lane, author of "Iridology". It will be noticed that there is in the outer rim of the iris a broad white ring and a narrow inner ring. These signs were produced by inorganic sodium which for several years I had taken in large quantities to neutralize a hyperacid condition of the stomach. Today, as a result of natural living and treatment, these sodium rings as well as many other drug signs have almost entirely disappeared, as shown in Fig.16. The crosses in Fig.15 indicate large iodine spots in the liver and right kidney as they appeared sixteen years ago. When I was a child our family physician had coated my neck at different times with iodine for the absorption of enlarged lymphatic glands. The poison had been absorbed throught the skin and had accumulated in liver and kidney. This, together with decidedly unnatural habits of living, produced chronic ailments which incidentally led me into the work I am doing now. Natural living and treatment have eliminated most of the sodium, as indicated in Fig.16, but today, after forty-five years, the iodine spots are still faintly visible in several places, namely in the left kidney, left lung and bronchi, and in right kidney and gall bladder.

RIGHT   LEFT

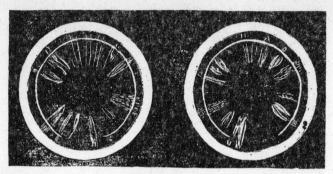

Fig. 15. Dr. Lane's Illustration Showing Appearance of Author's Eyes Sixteen Years Ago.

This proves that sodium and iodine, although congenial to the
human body in the organic form, cannot be taken with
impunity in the inorganic mineral form. The history of my
own case, as illustrated in these charts of the iris, shows that
sodium is much more easily and quickly eliminated from the
system than iodine. In this way iridology answers the question, "How long does it take to eliminate foreign matter and
poisons from the system?"

We have observed that the symptoms of drug poisoning
usually disappear much earlier than do the signs from the iris.
The apparent contradiction can be accounted for by the fact
that under the influence of natural living and treatment the
general constitutional conditions are so improved that,
although some of the poison is still present, the stonger
organs are now able to compensate for the deficiency on the

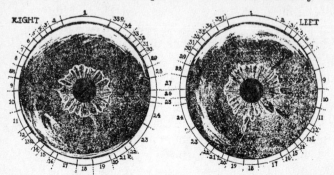

Fig. 16. The Author's Eyes at Present.

part of the weaker ones and therefore the effects of the drug
poisons are more readily eliminated from vital organs than
from the iris, on account of the more active metabolism in the
former. As regards signs of those minerals and earthy substances which are naturally present in the human body, we
find that iron, sodium, lime, sulphur and magnesium disappear much more quickly from the iris than iodine and
phosphorus, indicating that the latter are more destructive
and more difficult to dislodge (see also Chapter XXIV,
Basic Diagnosis).

Potassium (Kalium, K), Lime (Calcium, Ca), Magnesium (Mg)

Inorganic lime, magnesium and potassium show in the outer
margin of the iris in the form of a greyish white wreath somewhat similar to sodium (Colour plate, Figs a and c). Only
recently I examined a patient who came to us for diagnosis
and treatment from far-away New Mexico. His iris exhibited
very heavy sodium rings similar to my own as represented in
Fig.15. Quizzing at first failed to reveal the source of the
mineral accumulation in his system. Finally, however, it
became apparent that the sign in the iris must have been produced by drinking for many years the water from the shallow
wells of his native plains, strongly impregnated with alkali.
These signs gradually disappear from the iris when the
patient abstains from the use of mineral waters and adopts
eliminative diet and treatment.

    In the light of nature's records in the iris, it is little less
than criminal to give inorganic lime water, baking soda, iron,
magnesium and table salt to little babies in artificial food mix-
tures when good cow's milk and fruit juices contain these
minerals in great abundance in the live, organic (vitamin)
form. In the organic form in fruit juices and raw vegetable
extracts, all these minerals may be taken continually in large
quantities and will not show in the iris. An excess is easily
eliminated from the system through the excretory organs, and
we may safely say that the organism does not contain an
excess of these positive mineral elements until a point is
reached where the reaction of the urine is natural.

    Thus nature's records in the iris prove conclusively that

she does not intend us to use these elements in the inorganic
mineral form. The only apparent exception to this rule seems
to be sodium chloride, our common table salt. This might be
explained by the fact that sodium chloride is one of the
ordinary products of kidney elimination, while other sodium
combinations are not. There is no reason, however, why we
should endanger health by using table salt in such enormous
quantities as is customary, since we can supply the demand of
the system for sodium chloride in the organic form by adding
a liberal quantity of fruits and vegetables to our diet. There is
no doubt whatever that table salt, when taken habitually and
in considerable quantities, is very injurious to the system. The
reasons for and against the use of salt have been fully discussed in Vol.III of this series.

Sulphur (S)
(Colour Plate, Fig.d)

Sulphur, taken in the inorganic form, shows in the iris in the
area of stomach and intestines in the yellow sulphur colour.
After absorption it has at first a stimulating effect upon these
organs, but this is gradually followed by a sluggish atrophic
condition. Sometimes it is difficult to distinguish the sulphur
colour from the yellow of quinine or the yellowish colour of
scrofulous elimination through the digestive organs.

CHAPTER XI

SIGNS OF POISONS
IN THE EYE

The mineral elements discussed in the previous chapter are normally present in animal and human bodies and therefore are not poisonous in themselves unless ingested in the inorganic mineral form. There are, however, many inorganic or organic substances so inimical to health and life that nature never designed either animal or human bodies to receive them as foods or medicine. They are always poisonous to the system, even when taken in small quantities, and have a strong tendency to accumulate in parts and organs for which they exhibit particular affinity. Their presence and location is shown in the iris by well defined signs and discolourations as presented in the colour plate. I shall describe some of the best known and most widely used of these poisons, their signs in the iris and their effect upon the system.

Difficulties the Iridologist Must Meet
In the majority of cases the iris plainly displays signs of poisonous substances. However, when the diagnostician describes these poisons in the iris, the patient frequently denies with vehemence ever having taken "anything of the kind". He is unmindful of the following facts: First, that poisons are absorbed and thereafter remain indefinitely in certain parts of the system unless eliminated by radical methods. Secondly, that in the treatment of some "trifling children's disease", frequently enough poisons are given to affect the vital organs

and the iris for life. Thirdly, that poisons may be absorbed not only from patent medicines and remedies prescribed by physicians, but in various other ways, as lead from water pipes and glassware, from paints and printer's type; mercury in mines, smelters, mirror factories and from cosmetics; arsenic from green colours, wall paper, stuffed animals, etc. Almost every known poison is now used extensively in the arts and industries and in the preparation of multitudinous foods and other articles for daily use.

Reports of government chemists in Washington, whose duty is to examine food products for purity and quality, reveal astonishing conditions. They show that almost every kind of food for sale in grocery and market is contaminated or adulterated with deleterious substances, inorganic minerals, aniline dyes and various sorts of chemicals and poisons. Comments like the following by Dr. Wiley are common in magazines and the daily press, and are of interest in this connection: "Professor Wiley's reference was particularly to the aniline dyes derived from coal tar, which are used in colouring jellies and wines, as well as a great number of other food products and drinkables. Not long ago the Bureau of Chemistry dyed experimentally a number of pieces of white silk with chemical colours obtained from various liquors and articles of diet put up for commercial purposes. Preserved cherries, utilized in this manner, furnished a yard of pink silk; currant jam a yard of salmon silk; port wine a yard of purple silk; Burgundy wine a yard of magenta silk, tomato catsup a yard of light red silk, etc. The 'rosaline' used for colouring corned beef and sausage gave a dye of a beautiful and brilliant red. But in this line nothing has been found so suggestive of the rainbow as soda water syrups, which, taken in a bunch, are a chemical polychrome. The cheap candies which children buy are often most deleterious, containing clay, arsenic, sulphate of copper, and even prussic acid. Also they are coloured with the deadly aniline dyes. Many of the cheaper brands of chocolate on the market are composed mainly of starch and animal fat. They do not taste much like chocolate, but they easily pass for it, with the addition of oxide of iron — that is to say iron rust — to give the requisite colour. One plate of cheap ice cream analysed at the Bureau of Chemistry was found to contain as much fusel oil as five glasses of bad whisky. Of strawberry flavour, or what passed as such, it was in truth a chemical compound. A medicinal dose of sulphate of copper is three grains. Eat three small, artificially greened pickles, and you will get an equal quantity of this dangerous chemical. The salts of copper and zinc are commonly employed to give a green colour to peas, beans and other vegetables preserved for market in cans or glass jars."

Reports like the foregoing explain how certain poison signs may appear in the iris, even when the victim is unaware of "ever having taken such things".

Many people believe that the passage of the Pure Food Law has done away with wholesale food poisoning. They are seriously mistaken. All that the Pure Food Law prohibits is the use of poisonous substances in quantities large enough to injure the human body immediately. The law does not take into consideration the fact that the destructive effects may be cumulative and remote. In this respect the government falls into the same error as the medical profession. This is not to be wondered at since representatives of the allopathic school of medicine have assisted in framing these laws. A single dose of a certain drug poison given as medicine or used as a food preservative may not be harmful, but these poisons, as proved by the records of the iris, have a tendency to accumulate in the system in certain parts or organs for which they exhibit a special affinity. Therefore many small consecutive doses of poisonous medicines or food preservatives or adulterants will in time produce the effect of a big dose. This explains the presence of the signs of boric acid salicylites, copper, lead, zinc, coal tar poisons, etc., in the eyes of people who "do not know of ever having taken these things".

Doctors Don't Believe in Giving Strong Medicines.

Some time ago in a public clinic I detected in the iris of a young man the evidences of strychnine, iodine, quinine and mercury. He strenuously denied having taken so many poisons. "My doctor," said he, "does not believe in giving strong medicines, and I am sure I have never taken all that stuff." I asked him to bring to the next clinic some of his doctor's prescriptions. A few days later he complied with the request and brought two of the most recent ones. Both contained three of the poisons which the diagnosis had revealed in the iris. Of course he had taken the same drugs many years ago; otherwise they would not have shown in the iris at the time of the diagnosis.

Records in the Iris More Reliable Than Memory.

The following incident illustrates that the records in the iris are frequently more reliable than the memory of the patient. Several years ago an elderly woman came for diagnosis and treatment. The outer margin of her iris showed distinctly the whitish flakes of arsenic (Colour plate, Fig.b) and in the left cerebrum a heavy red blotch of iodine. Referring to the signs of arsenic, I said to her, "You suffer with severe pains all over your body and your muscles are sensitive to touch." She acknowledged that "rheumatism" and multiple neuritis had for many years been the curse of her life. Referring to the iodine spot in the left brain, I continued my diagnosis: "You must have had severe chronic left side headaches." This she also confirmed. For twenty years she had never been free from an excruciating headache; as she expressed it, "It often seemed my head would split in two." Naturally she wished to learn the cause of her long continued suffering, but when I informed her that arsenic and iodine were responsible for her "rheumatism" and chronic headaches, she denied ever having taken these drugs. "In my younger years," she said, "before these ailments developed, I was a strong, healthy girl and never took medicines of any kind. How could arsenic and iodine have caused these troubles?"

A few weeks later, however, in consultation she inadvertently remarked that her husband, who was a musician, employed his leisure hours by stuffing the skins of wild animals. "Did he use arsenic in his taxidermic work?" I asked. "Oh, yes," she answered. "He often explained to me that his animals were so well preserved because he used large quantities of arsenic in their preparation." "Did he have many of these animals around the house?" "They were in the parlour, sitting room and in the bed-rooms." Noticing my smile, she added, "I can see now where the arsenic and the 'rheumatism' came from." I then continued, "Now, let us find out where the iodine came from." Her interest in the diagnosis now being thoroughly aroused she thought back over the past for a few months and then exclaimed, "How could I have forgotten? Twenty-five years ago, when a servant in Berlin, I accidentally hurt my knee. A painful swelling followed. The cook told me to go into her room and take some medicine that had cured her rheumatism and would be just the thing for my knee. Acting on the suggestion, I took a good swallow from the cook's bottle. That was the last I remembered for several days. When I regained consciousness I was told that the medicine was a stong preparation of iodine for external use only."

Latin Names to Cover Ignorance.
Prospective patients expect to hear from us the same old familiar Greek and Latin names which they have heard from other doctors, professors and specialists. If the diagnostician of the iris fails to employ the same familiar terms, they are sceptical of the diagnosis. Suppose a doctor, listening to a patient who describes his changing aches and pains should say to him, "My dear sir, you suffer from moving pains," the patient would answer indignantly, "I know that myself; I want to know what my disease is." If the doctor tells him he has "rheumatism", which in English means nothing more nor less than "moving pains", his client is perfectly satisfied, pays his fee and goes home well pleased that he now knows what ails him. He has "rheumatism".

Several weeks ago a woman came to me for diagnosis. The iris revealed the greenish wreath of mercury in the regions of the brain and spinal cord. The areas of the stomach, bowels and liver were dark brown. The following conversation took place: "For many years you have been suffering from indigestion, chronic constipation and sluggishness of the liver. To better the condition you have taken a great deal of calomel." "It is the only way I can keep my bowels open and my liver active." "Of late years you have had shooting pains in the back, the lower limbs and around the stomach. The calomel, which is mercury, is causing inflammation of the spinal cord." The woman confirmed every symptom revealed by the records in the eyes, but did not return for treatment. Several days later a friend of hers informed me that she was not at all satisfied because I had failed to tell her she had rheumatism. "Every other doctor has told me I have rheumatism," she complained, "and if the diagnosis from the iris cannot show that much it is not to be relied upon." As a matter of fact she is in the advanced stages of locomotor ataxia.

Not All Conditions in the Body Visible in the Iris.

As before stated, not all poisons taken, injuries sustained, nor all pathological lesions show in the iris. Many times we are disappointed by not finding the lesions we expect and are looking for. Drug poisons may be eliminated from the system in some cases more than in others. Individuals differ greatly in drug tolerance. That is, some eliminate certain poisons very readily and very thoroughly while others are permanently affected by even small doses. Hahnemann, speaking of mercury, said, "Some people are so susceptible to this drug that even a few doses of it will make them 'weather prophets' for life." Iridology is a comparatively new science and many things about it remain to be discovered and to be explained. We do claim, however, that the well proven facts which we already possess are sufficient to make this new science of immense value to the diagnostician and the physician.

Alteratives.

Mercury, iodine and arsenic are the principal alteratives. The multitudinous preparations of these drugs are used by the allopathic school principally in the treatment of syphilis. Should you ask a doctor how these drugs cure disease, if truthful he would have to answer, "We do not know." Sajous tries to explain the action of mercury and other alteratives by saying they stimulate the activity of the ductless glands. For this assertion, however, he cannot produce the slightest proof. A medical dictionary which I have before me gives the following definition: "Alteratives are certain remedies that alter the course of morbid conditions in some way not yet understood, perhaps by promoting metabolism. We know, for instance, that mercury cures syphilitis sores or arsenic chronic skin diseases, but we do not know how or why."

The solution of the problem seems so obvious that it is
hard to understand how and why it has baffled medical
science for so long. The fundamental law of cure will help us
to solve the mystery. According to this law all acute diseases
are the result of nature's efforts to expel inner latent morbid
encumbrances. In other words, acute diseases represent
increased and specialized activity of vital force. When we
introduce into the system, in the form of mercury, iodine or
arsenic, a stronger and more dangerous enemy than the constitutional disease taint which nature is trying to eliminate,
then the healing forces, like good tacticians, leave the weaker
foe for a time and turn to repel the new and more dangerous
invader. A man attacked by a child defends himself, but when
confronted by a powerful adult, turns from the weaker foe to
the stronger. Similarly the healing forces of the human
organism turn from their fight against the stronger drug
poison. The disease taints recede into the system, the surface
symptoms disappear, the patient thinks he is cured, but the
doctor knows better because in the medical college he has
been taught "Never guarantee a cure."

After a while nature may reassert herself and make
another attempt to eliminate the disease poisons. Again and
again her benevolent efforts are suppressed until the entire
organism is saturated with mercury or other alteratives to the
point where vital force, weakened and defeated in every quarter, can no longer react against the disease taints. This process of progressive poisoning may have to be maintained for
two or three years before vital force is effectually defeated
and bound; then the patient is told he "may now safely
marry." But what is the real state of affairs? The outward
manifestations of healing activity, the scrofulous, syphilitic
or tuberculous sores, the itch or eczema have disappeared
from the surface, but these disorders are by no means cured.
On their retreat into the interior, the danger from the disease
taints is always great and it often happens that they invade
and destroy vital parts and organs. The external discharge or
ulcer may become internal tuberculosis or cancer.

CHAPTER XII

MERCURY HYDRARGYRUM OR QUICKSILVER
(Colour Plate, Figs.c and f)

These are the three names for the only liquid metallic element. It is used as medicine in more than a hundred different forms. The nitrates, oxides, chlorides and iodides are the salts most commonly employed in medicine. Other preparations commonly used are blue mass and calomel, and in syphilis the bichloride, the yellow iodide and the red iodide. Still other preparations are cyanide, the yellow sub sulphate, mercury and chalk, the plaster and the iodide of mercury and arsenic, yellow wash, black wash, corrosive sublimate, etc.

Effect of the Drug from the Viewpoint of Natural Therapeutics.
In the first few years, after the mercury has been absorbed by the organism, and while it is still wandering in the circulation and in the tissues, it shows in the iris, especially in the upper half, as a whitish film. After five or more years it begins to condense into a greenish crescent of metallic lustre on the uppermost margin of the brain region in the blue eye and of a bluish colour in the brown eye. In serious cases this greenish rim may extend all around the outer margin of the iris. The metal, on account of its deteriorating effect upon the skin, also greatly broadens and intensifies the scurf rim (Colour plate, Fig.d). It takes this treacherous, insidious poison from five to fifteen years to create its havoc in the brain and ner-

vous system. When this commences, unless radical measures
are employed, it marks the beginning of the end — the
development of locomotor ataxia, paralysis agitans,
paresis, etc.

The first and secondary stages of syphilis mark nature's
efforts to expel the syphilitic virus; the tertiary stage is due to
the destructive effects of mercury, iodine, potassium, salvarsan (arsenic), etc., on the brain, spinal cord and other vital
organs. "All wrong," says the allopath, "these tertiary
symptoms are due to syphilis, not to mercury." To this we
answer, "Not so; we have treated hundreds of cases of luetic
diseases but not a single one has ever developed any tertiary
symptoms. . ." Syphilitic cases under favourable circumstances recover under homoeopathic or Christian Science treatment. If the highly diluted remedy or the metaphysical
formula does not actually cure the disease, it at least does not
interfers with nature's cleansing, healing processes. Treatment under our system usually lasts from three to six months
and after this natural cure the patient's system is purer than
before infection because the ulcers, discharges or skin eruptions have acted as fontanelles and the treatment has
eliminated not only the venereal virus, but also other
hereditary and acquired traits latent in the system. On the
other hand, we have in every case of locomotor ataxia,
paralysis agitans or paresis, unravelled a history of some
form of alterative treatment and usually found the corresponding signs of these poisons in the iris.

The allopath says, "All this talk does not amount to anything; it is unorthodox and unscientific; all our authorities
contradict it." This possibly may be so; but the experiences of
thousands of patients, for twenty to thirty years slowly tor-
tured to death, verifies our contention. Not even the fanatical
inquisition nor the imaginative brain of a cruel savage has
ever invented tortures more inhuman and devastating than
those inflicted by the "alteratives". How much more merciful
would it be to give these victims of medical malpractice in the
beginning a good dose of an "alterative" and have done with
it. When you see vigorous, blue eyed manhood succumb in
the prime of life to destructive diseases "which have never
before been in the family" — think of the alteratives. When

you see a young wife, once the embodiment of health, fading away after marriage, a victim of mysterious ailments — think of the alteratives. Medical authorities claim that over fifty per cent of all men in large cities have been treated for venereal diseases. When you see the offspring of a healthy mother made defective by scrofula, chronic catarrh, decayed teeth, epilepsy or idiocy — think of the alteratives. Anaemia, rachitis and scrofulous constitutions in children are only too often due to the poisoned blood of their progenitors. With every additional year of practice and observation my conviction is strengthened that drug poisoning is the most fruitful source of chronic and hereditary disease. Nature tries to remedy the effects of wrong living by acute reactions of brief duration, but three fourths of the most dreadful cases of chronic disease coming to us for diagnosis and treatment are caused by the suppression of nature's acute healing efforts and by the destructive effects of poisonous drugs, vaccines, serums, antitoxins, and of uncalled for surgical operations.

Locomotor ataxia, paralysis agitans and paresis are man made. Nature never punishes and curses her children in such a dreadful manner. All such suffering is the result of human ignorance, prejudice and indifference. Lest these statements appear exaggerated and iconoclastic, I shall quote passages from allopathic authorities who consciously or unwittingly confirm my position. A Ross Diefendorf, M.D., is an authority on mental disease in this country. He was formerly lecturer on Psychiatry at Yale University and a member of many medical societies. His book "Clinical Psychiatry" is in common use as a text-book in many American colleges. It is interesting to note how unconsciously he confirms our claims that mercury and not syphilis is to blame for the entire train of so called syphilitic symptoms. In Chapter VI of his work he has this to say on the subject of Dementia Paralytica (paresis).

"Dementia Paralytica, or general paresis of the insane, is a chronic psychosis of middle age, characterized by progressive mental deterioration with symptoms of excitation of the central nervous system, leading to absolute dementia and paralysis, and pathologically, by a fairly definite series of organic changes in the brain and spinal cord, probably the result of some toxin, in the origin of which syphilis is most often an important factor.

"Aetiolgy — The disease is unknown among the uncivilized nations and is most prevalent in western Europe and North America, hence, it seems to be a disease of modern civilization. In America, the disease comprises from five to eight percent of the admissions to insane institutions, but in some European cities, notably Berlin and Munich, the paretics average thirty-six to forty-five percent of the male admissions. The disease is somewhat more prevalent in large cities and manufacturing centres, whilst it is relatively rare in farming communities."

Uncivilized nations do not treat syphilis or other diseases with mercury; therefore, we find among them no Dementia Paralytica, locomotor ataxia or paralysis agitans. These diseases are found only in localities of the earth where drug stores flourish. Therefore, paralytic diseases are more prevalent in large cities and manufacturing centres where syphilitic diseases and consequent mercurial treatment are more prevalent. Again to quote Dr. Diefendorf, he says:

"Negresses show a striking tendency to the disease; in Connecticut the negress paretics are ten times more prevalent that the female white paretics."

If negroes are free from the disease in Africa, as medical authorities state, but "show a striking tendency" to it in civilized countries, how can this be explained except on the ground that the disease is the product of unnatural treatment and drug poisoning? To quote again:

"Our average age of onset in 172 cases is forty-two years. Kraepelin in 249 cases finds that it occurs preeminently in middle life, as eighty-one percent of the cases occur between thirty and fifty years, the disease rarely appearing before twenty-five or after fifty-five years of age."

Syphilitic diseases are usually contracted between the ages of twenty and thirty and it takes from ten to twenty years for mercury to complete its work of destruction in brain and nerve matter. To quote again:

"Recently a number of cases of juvenile paresis have been reported occurring between the ages of ten to twenty years, in which hereditary paresis, syphilis and alcoholism are prominent factors. Clinically, the juvenile form is characterized by simple deterioration of three or four years' duration with numerous paralytic attacks, choreic disturbances, and paralyses."

Frequently young children are subjected to prolonged mercurial treatment on the mere suspicion that they have hereditary syphilis, or for curing eczemata. Scenes like the following are of almost daily occurrence in medical clinics. A mother enters the clinic with a child whose body is covered with skin eruptions. One professor says the disease is of a scrofulous nature, another calls it eczema, another hereditary syphilis. The mother denies that the latter disease has ever been in the family. The professor tells the students: "You can never believe syphilitics, they always lie." "We can easily find out whether this eruption is of a syphilitic nature or not. Put the patient for six months under mercurial treatment and if the eruptions permanently disappear, then the case is syphilitic." Thus hundreds of people, including children, in civilized countries are innocently subjected to the horrible suffering incidental to mercurial poisoning without ever having contracted venereal diseases.

Another large percentage of paralytic and paretic patients have accumulated the mercury in the guise of liver and bowel tonics (calomel) and antiseptics. Dr. Diefendorf says:

"The disease afflicts chiefly the unmarried, and among the women especially prostitutes; in our experience prostitutes are forty-five percent more prone to the disease than other women.

"Among the causes of the disease, syphilis is statistically the most prominent. Its prevalence varies, according to various authors, from one to six tenths percent, but most observers place it between thirty-four and sixty-five percent."

"The character of the toxin and the source from which it arises are questions still in doubt. Syphilis cannot be the sole cause of paresis, as long as it does not exist in more than thirty-four to sixty-five percent of the cases.

Furthermore, paresis, anatomically, is not a simple syphilitic process. Again the late manifestations of syphilis arise within a comparatively short time after primary symptoms, while paresis does not develop until ten or more years have elapsed after the initial lesion."

No, syphilis is not the sole cause of paralytic and paretic diseases and the character of the toxin from which they arise is not in doubt — it is mercury or some other alterative. This is exactly what I have always maintained. Syphilis is an acute infectious disease, which under right treatment runs its natural course within a comparatively short time, never to appear again unless a new infection has taken place. On the other hand, the history of people who never had syphilis, but who were poisoned by mercury in mine or factory, proves that it takes from ten to fifteen years before the poison exhibits its worst effects.

Professor E.A. Farrington, one of the most celebrated homoeopathic physicians of the nineteenth century, says concerning the destructive after effects of mercury, of which homoeopaths have made careful study (Clinical Materia Medica):

"The more remote symptoms of mercurial poisoning are these. You will find that the blood becomes impoverished. The albumin and fibrin of that fluid are affected. They are diminished, and you find in their place a certain fatty substance, the composition of which I do not exactly know. Consequently, as a prominent symptom, the body wastes and emaciates. The patient suffers from fever, which is rather hectic in its character. The periostium becomes affected, and you then have a characteristic group of mercury pains, bone pains worse in the changes of the weather, worse in the warmth of the bed, and chilliness with and after stool. The skin becomes rather of a brownish hue; ulcers form, particularly on the legs; they are stubborn and will not heal. The patient is troubled with sleeplessness and ebullitions of blood at night; he is hot and cannot sleep; he is thrown quickly into a perspiration, which perspiration gives him no relief

"The entire system suffers also, and you have here two

series of symptoms. At first the patient becomes anxious and restless and cannot remain quiet, he changes his position; he moves about from place to place; he seems to have a great deal of anxiety about the heart, praecordial anguish, as it is termed, particularly at night.

"Then, in another series of symptoms, there are jerkings of the limbs, making the patient appear as though he were attacked by St. Vitus' dance. Or, you may notice what is more common yet, trembling of the hands, this tremor being altogether beyond the control of the patient and gradually spreading over the entire body, giving you a resemblance to paralysis agitans or shaking palsy.

"Finally, the patient becomes paralysed, cannot move his limbs, his mind becomes lost, and he presents a perfect picture of imbecility. He does all sorts of queer things. He sits in the corner with an idiotic smile on his face, playing with straws; he is forgetful, cannot remember even the most ordinary events. He becomes disgustingly filthy and eats his own excrement. In fact, he is a perfect idiot.

"Be careful how you give mercury; it is a treacherous medicine. It seems often indicated. You give it and relieve; but your patient is worse again in a few weeks, and then you give it again with relief. By and by, it fails you. Now, if I want to make a permanent cure, for instance, in a scrofulous child, I will very seldom give him mercury; should I do so, it will at least be only as an intercurrent remedy."

Dr. Hermann, of Vienna, has written several books in which he proves that syphilis is not a constitutional disease, that under hygienic living and treatment it is self limited, that it runs its regular natural course and when properly treated never produces any tertiary symptoms. This I, myself, have proved in hundreds of cases. It is impossible to quote better authority for these facts than Dr. Hermann. For thirty years he was superintendent of the syphilitic wards in the Hospital Wieden, near Vienna, one of the greatest institutions in the world for the treatment of luetic ailments. He claims that during the thirty years of his incumbency he treated sixty thousand cases of syphilitic diseases without the use of mercury

and that not in a single case thus treated and cured did he
observe a spontaneous recurrence, an exhibition of tertiary
symptoms or hereditary transmission. His work was done in a
municipal institution to which the doctors and students of
Vienna had free access, and thus was constantly under the
scrutiny of the great medical schools of Vienna. I take the
liberty of translating some interesting passages from his
book: "Es giebt keine consitutionelle syphilis" — "Syphilis is
not a constitutional disease".

"Syphilis is as old as humanity. Its peculiar symptoms
are described in the Third Book of Moses; the disease
was well known to Hippocrates and Celsus and is
minutely described by Tremelius and Beza as well as by
many other writers of subsequent centuries. After the
discovery of America, diseases of this type were found,
in exactly the same form as we know them today, among
the Indians. At the end of the fifteenth century they
appeared as discharge or ulcer, with or without following figwarts (condyloma), inflammation of the glands
and skin eruptions. These always appear in direct
organic connection with one of the original lesions. Until
then syphilis was looked upon as a simple local disease
which ran its natural course without affecting the
organism as a whole. It was thoroughly cured by
hygienic, natural methods of treatment. There were no
tertiary symptoms nor transmission to offspring. All the
old physicians held this opinion; this is proved by the
fact that up to the end of the fifteenth century constitutional syphilis is nowhere mentioned or described.
In 1786 Hunter first spoke of its local and constitutional
forms. He described the hard chancre as a symptom of
the malignant form and originated the idea of constitutional syphilis. Ulcers of the mucous membranes,
skin eruptions, inflammations of the iris and of the bones
were classed by him as secondary symptoms. The later
affections of the inner organs, of the liver, kidneys,
heart, lungs, brain, nerves and blood vessels, hair and
nails were looked upon as tertiary and quarternary
forms.

In view of these teachings of the regular school, the

question arises: is the syphilis of former centuries
another disease than the one we know? Is modern
syphilis a new disease, unknown to the ancients, or were
they lacking in diagnostic ability, since they did not suspect the existence of the constitutional disease?
The ancient physicians were right. Syphilis, originating
in the human organism, is undoubtedly the same disease
now as then. It has not changed its origin and has always
run its natural course without transgressing natural
limits. The physicians of antiquity observed conscien-
tiously and with understanding the course of the disease
and treated it rationally, as a local ailment which never
affected the organism as a whole."
These expositions of Dr. Hermann I can fully confirm.
Of the hundreds of cases of syphilis and gonorrhoea which
have been treated by us from their inception (before any form
of suppressive treatment had been applied), not a single one
has developed constitutional symptoms of hereditary tendencies. Our natural methods of treatment purify the system
from within, allow the disease to run its natural course,
unhindered and unchecked. When, under such treatment discharges, ulcers, inflammations and eruptions disappear, the
organism is as pure as before infection, if not more pure. We
say this advisedly; the natural process of elimination removes
not only the disease virus but other hereditary and acquired
taints as well. Dr. Hermann continues:
"The disease conditions usually diagnosed as constitutional syphilis are the results of mercurial treatment
or of other disease taints in the body. This I prove, first
by clinical observation of the natural course of the disease, and second by the positive chemical proof of the
presence of mercury in the system. We have found the
mercury in the ashes of the bones of mercurial patients.
A patient is coming to us now who went through a course
of mercurial treatment two years ago. The gold rings on
his fingers turn black under the effect of the mercury
which his system is now eliminating. Among the thousands of luetics whom for thirty years I observed in the
Hospital Wieden in Vienna and who were treated
without mercury, not a single one developed con-

stitutional syphilis. Cases of so called constitutional syphilis that came to us suffering with ulcerations of the palate, mouth and nose, with bone pain, gummata of the brain and inflammation of the nerves, all had histories of mercurial treatment. Hundreds of electolytical analyses of urine, sputum, persipiration, blood and other body materials revealed the presence of mercury, while a comparatively small percentage exhibited scrofulous or tuberculous symptoms. Thus it became clear to me that the entire chain of symptoms which are commonly diagnosed as constitutional syphilis are nothing but the effects of mercury in the human body. Workers salivated in the mercury mines in Idria, who never suffered with syphilis, exhibit all the symptoms of so called secondary and tertiary syphilis. In the blood and urine of all these patients I also found mercury. In fact, the various forms of mercurialism everywhere occur among people who continually come in contact with mercury and thus absorb it; no age, no sex is immune. This is verified by physicians practicing among quicksilver miners, mirror, thermometer and barometer makers, etc. For these reasons chronic mercurialism is always prevalent in localities where, by physicians and laymen, syphilis is treated by mercury. Mercurialism is very common on the coast of the Adriatic, the Ost and North Sea and the Mediterranean because in these countries quicksilver in its various forms is in common use as a universal home remedy. In large inland cities and sea ports, chronic mercurialism is much more prevalent than in country districts, because, in the former, syphilis and its mercurial treatment are much more common than in the latter. The question naturally arises why, in spite of strictly scientific proof and of extraordinary practical results, these very teachings are not generally accepted and why the regular school has not examined officially my theory and treatment. The answer is evident. Ancient systems of medicine with all their errors, assumptions, superstitions and prejudices, are deeply rooted in medical science. The schools, blindly worshipping authority, have strenuously opposed strictly scientific investiga-

tions. The natural treatment of syphilis brings light into
the dark labyrinth of the old system, destroys the nimbus
of old school wisdom and the idol worship of the quicksilver treatment. The world resents nothing so deeply
and punishes so harshly as the uprooting of dear old
superstitions; therefore the bitter opposition of the
regular school to my teachings and my practice.

What wonder that my enemies, in fanatical zeal, tried to
oust me from my stronghold in the Hospital Wieden,
when Dr. Hebra, according to his own confession
wished: 'That the hospital might be blown into the
air.'

In 1867, by means of unjust accusations, my enemies
succeeded in procuring a government investigation of
my work and my institution. In 1868, however, their
machinations met with miserable defeat, for Dr. Hebra,
the head of the commission appointed to investigate my
methods, had to admit in his official report: "That the
government could sustain no objection against the anti-
mercurial treatment of syphilis in the Hospital Wieden.'
In justification of their own methods he added: 'Syphilis
is curable without mercury but we give it because it cures
the disease quicker and because it is harmless.' "

Later Dr. Hermann goes on to say:

"Finally I retired, firmly hoping that for some time at
least my methods of treatment, eminently successful for
thirty years, would be maintained. But this last and fer-
vent desire of my declining days was not to be fulfilled.
In the holy place where, for a lifetime I battled bravely
against the abuses of mercurialism the altars devoted to
the fetish quicksilver are now restored. The quacks and
charletans will again exploit the blind, foolish and
superstitious masses and will again endanger and destroy the public health; syphilis will reappear in the horrible forms so common thirty years ago. The people
themselves, realizing the terrible effects of mercurialism, must energetically oppose the false teachings
of the schools, must bear witness to the truth and protect
their bodies against contamination with the vile poison.
In recognition of the fact that the mercurial treatment

practised by the schools endangers not only the individual but society at large, through its weakening and
degenerating influences on our people, and especially on
the younger generation, it is the duty of the government,
legally to exclude mercury from medical practice.

Thus wrote Dr. Hermann, a graduate of the great medical schools in Vienna, but the work of mercurial poisoning
goes merrily on until the insane asylums and homes for incur-
ables can no longer take care of the harvest. Poisonous drugs
destroy brain and nerve matter and alcohol is often made the
scapegoat. Look closer, gentlemen, and you will find that in
many cases alcoholism is an effect rather than a cause. The
diagnosis from the eye fully confirms our estimate of the true
nature of the different stages of syphilis.

If syphilis in itself were a chronic constitutional disease,
like scrofula or psora, it would exhibit its presence in the body
by a special sign, but it appears in the iris only under the common signs of acute and chronic catarrhal conditions. On the
other hand, cures diagnosed and treated by the regular profession as secondary or tertiary syphilis exhibit the signs of me
cury, iodine, potassium and arsenic (Salvarsan). A few years
ago salvarsan was heralded as a positive cure for syphilis.
Now, already (1918), medical authorities admit that the
poison is not coming up to expectations, for everywhere they
now combine the ancient mercurial and potassium iodide
treatment with the salvarsan. The principle difference between salvarsan and mercury is that the former is more quickly destructive. Neither is curative.

A Typical Case.

A few years ago a man about forty years of age came to us in a
pitiable condition afflicted with locomotor ataxia. Every doctor he had consulted was positive that he was suffering from
tertiary syphilis. The Wasserman and Noguchi tests always
proved "positive". Still the patient, as well as his mother and
wife, denied strenuously that he was ever infected with
venereal disease. The doctors of course were convinced that it
was another case of "syphilitic liar" (See colour plate, Fig. f).
On examination I found in the iris well defined signs of mercury and I tried to find where and in what form Mr. K. had

absorbed the poison. The mother admitted that she had been
in the habit of giving calomel to her children, but I could hardly believe that this alone accounted for his terrible condition.
Several months after I had made my first examination the
wife of the patient came to me and said "Doctor, we know
now where my husband got the mercury. When he was fourteen years of age his mother put him to work in the Pullman
car shops. He was given employment in the mirror depart-
ment and there he silvered mirrors for two years." The
"silver" on mirrors consists largely of quicksilver. The lad
undoubtedly absorbed the mercury through the skin and
through inhalation. The poison began to show its destructive
effects when he was about twenty-five years of age. At forty
he was in the advanced stages of locomotor ataxia. This case,
like many others, also proves that the Wasserman and
Noguchi tests show "positive" in mercurial and other forms of
mineral poisoning as well as in syphilis. Many patients are
thus wrongly accused of being syphilitic because the doctors
do not know how to differentiate between venereal diseases
and drug poisoning. Such unjust accusations have frequently
caused great humiliation, domestic troubles and divorce pro-
ceedings. The unfortunate victim of medical malpractice is
thus robbed not only of his health but also of his moral
reputation.

The Treatment of Mercurialism.

Mercurialism is easily cured while the poison is still diffuse in
the system, but its elimination becomes more difficult when it
is concentrated in the brain and spinal cord as indicated by the
corresponding sign in the iris (Colour plate, Figs. e and f). But
many such cases well advanced in locomotor ataxia and
paralysis agitans have yielded to our natural treatment. One
such patient had had locomotor ataxia fully developed for six
years. When he came to us he had to take, according to his
own statement, a few dozen doses a day of some powerful
narcotic to subdue the "lightning" and "girdle pains". After
five months' treatment the pains had disappeared and he felt
well enough to quit treatment. One of my first patients, Mr. S.
was also a case of locomotor ataxia, fully developed for seven
years. He was past the painful and in the paralytic stage. He

could walk only with the aid of a crutch and stick. The
sphincters of the bladder and anus were partially paralysed so
that at times he could not control the movements of the
bowels and of the bladder. After seven months' treatment he
was able to work at the bench in a violin factory, and after
eighteen months he worked as a carpenter in the Pullman car
shops. When I met him a few years afterward he told me that
he continued to work during the hot summer when most of the
employees laid off on account of the unbearable heat. Such
cases of course require thorough systematic natural treatment
by all methods at our disposal. The curability of such a case
frequently can be determined only by giving these methods a
fair trial.

Deception Taught in Medical Schools.

In medical schools students are warned not to use the word
"calomel" in their prescriptions, "because people are afraid of
it". They are instructed to write instead "Hydrargyrum",
which is the Greek word for mercury. When the mother
pleads, "Doctor, I do not want you to give calomel to the
baby," she is shown that calomel does not appear on the prescription; she does not suspect that "hydrargarum" — Hg — is
the same thing. Why this deception? Because people look for
instantaneous results. The doctor who cannot produce them
loses his bread and butter. Homoeopathy and other natural
methods of treatment are not popular because they are regarded as "too slow". "Something must be done at once". The one
who can most quickly move the liver and the bowels, run
down the fever, suppress skin eruptions, ulcers and catarrhal
discharges is the best doctor. In their anxiety for the loved one
people will insist on "quick results".

Sometimes when sorely pressed in acute crises, even
those who thoroughly understand the teachings of Natural
Therapeutics succumb to fear and resort once more to drugs
in order to produce temporary relief. "I know you are right,
Doctor. I do not doubt the teachings of Natural Therapeutics,
but I cannot endure to look any longer on this suffering. We
will use the drugs just once more, and then stick to natural
methods all the closer in order to eliminate the after effects."
It is the old story — "I will sin just once more, and then I will

be good." But the "once more" is frequently once too often.
When nature under the influence of natural living and treatment has worked up to a healtng crisis, suppression is
dangerous and often fatal. The climax of a healing crisis
marks nature's supreme effort to overcome a diseased condition, and if at this critical moment she is thwarted again, the
healing forces of the system are not strong enough to overcome the new suppression, and a relapse into chronic disease
or death itself are the usual results.

It is the anxiety for immediate relief which keeps alive
the drug curse and which has turned homoeopathy into "mongrelism". I once attended a clinic presided over by a homeopathic physician. One of the subjects was a young man
suffering from venereal disease. After the diagnosis and
usual discussion of the case one of the students was ordered
by the professor to give the man a thorough mercurial inunction. I asked the doctor: "Is this homeopathic treatment?"
Smilingly he replied: "I suppose not; but these people want
quick results. If we do not produce them they will go to the
man on the next corner". This is also the excuse of the saloon
keeper for remaining in his line of business.

Information from Allopathic Sources.

The following description of mercury, as well as those of all
other drugs in this compilation, their uses and their chronic
effects upon the system, were compiled by our colleague, Dr.
Jean du Plessis from the latest standard works on materia
medica in the John Crerear Library. These data from
allopathic sources prove that the destructive effects of these
so called medicines are well known to the medical profession.

Mercury.

Allopathic Uses:
1. Caustic against luetic lesions and small skin growths.
2. Antiseptic dressing for wounds and ulcers.
3. Ringworm and other parasitic skin diseases.
4. Lues and chronic internal inflammations.
5. Alterative or intercurrent remedy.
6. Popular purgative in the form of calomel.

Accidental Poisoning:
1. Workmen handling mercury in mines, in the manufacture of thermometers, mirrors, etc.
2. Blue ointment. Grey salve.
3. Blue pills and other patent remedies for costiveness.
4. Amalgam tooth fillings.

Toxicology:
1. Circulates as oxyalbuminate of mercury, impoverishing both plasma and corpuscles. Soon leaves blood stream to enter tissues, where it may remain indefinitely.

Symptoms of Hydrargyrism or Chronic Mercurial Poisoning.
1. Salivation.
2. Loose teeth — extraction followed by ulceration of sockets.
3. Mercurial teeth of Hutchinson found in children suffering from congenital syphilis, or according to Natural Therapeutics, from congenital mercurialism.
4. Dyspepsia. Diarrhoea alternating with stubborn constipation — stools contain sulphide of mercury.
5. Mercurial eczema.
6. Ulcerations of mucous membranes and skin.
7. Softening of the bones, and pains in the same.
8. Peripheral neuritis — girdle pains radiating down the limbs.
9. Anaesthetic patches.
10. Descending tremor progressing from intermittent with excitement and exertion, to continuous during waking hours only.
11. Impaired reflexes followed by various forms of paralysis such as locomotor ataxia, paralysis agitans or paresis.

Elimination of Drug in Healing Crises.
Takes place through skin eruptions, furuncles, ulcers, abscesses, various forms of feverish and catarrhal processes, open sores and haemorrhoidal discharges.
Ordinary symptoms of "salivation" and metallic tastes in the mouth are frequent symptoms.
Dizziness, nervous and mental disturbances are of common occurrence.

Signs in the Iris.

While in the circulation it shows especially in the upper half of the iris as a whitish film. This, after five years or more, begins to condense into a greenish crescent of metallic lustre in the blue eye (Colour plate, Fig.c) and of bluish colour in the brown eye (Colour plate, Fig.f). The greenish crescent in serious cases may extend all round the outer margin of the iris. The scurf rim becomes broader and darker in colour.

How Dentists Contract Mercurial Poisoning.

A few days ago I examined the eyes of a patient which revealed the typical "mercurial iris" covered all over with a heavy whitish "felt-like" film. The outer margin of the iris was bordered by a heavy, black scurf rim. The scurf rim in turn was surrounded by the transparent bluish, greenish mercurial ring which encroaches upon the white (sclera) of the eyeball. The brain region showed the fine white crescent of destruction of brain matter, indicating paresis.

The patient denied having taken mercury in any form. After much quizzing he finally admitted that as a dentist he had for twenty-five years mixed the amalgam for tooth fillings in his bare hands. He is in advanced stage of paresis. This morning he tried to kill his wife.

CHAPTER XIII

CINCHONA — QUININE
(Colour Plate, Fig.c)

Cinchona or Peruvian bark was introduced into Europe as a medicinal remedy about the year 1820. Its best known alkaloid is quinine. Probably no drug has been more popular, both with the medical profession and the laity, than quinine. In many sections of the country especially those affected by catarrhal diseases or malarial fevers, the drug is taken as freely and regularly as an ordinary condiment. People are surprised when told that it is a powerful poison, and that when taken continuously, even in small doses, it will produce a variety of serious chronic ailments, such as indigestion, constipation, rheumatism and neuralgia, deafness, colour blindness and total blindness, irritability, neurasthenia and insanity. In consultaion with the doctor, patients are told that the drug is harmless, while the lecturer in classroom, and materia medica, describe in detail the cumulative effects of this and other poisonous agents. They picture with terrible realism the symptoms of chronic mercurialism, iodism, bromism, cinchonism, the cocaine, chloral and morphine habits, and then continue prescribing these drugs as though they were as innocent as bonbons.

The diagnosis from the iris brings proof positive of the cumulative and destructive effects of these agents. I have previously called attention to the fact that every substance poisonous to the human organism if taken repeatedly or in sufficient quantity, manifests in the iris by peculiar signs and colours easily recognized by the trained eye. These signs and colours diminish and disappear when the corresponding poisons are eliminated from the system, accompanied by their own peculiar crisis manifestations. This is proof that these poisonous drugs are not eliminated as quickly and thoroughly as the allopathic physician tries to make himself believe.

Next to iodine, the presence of quinine in the body is more readily recognised in the iris than that of any other poisonous substance. It shows as a yellowish discolouration, sometimes whitish and sometimes approaching in hue a reddish brown, according to the chemical combinations it has entered into. It shows particularly and most prominently in the brain, eyes, ears, stomach and bowels, indicating that it has a strong affinity for these parts and organs. In old malarial cases it also shows in the areas of liver and spleen.

When we see the signs of the drug in the iris of a patient we need only take any materia medica and read the typical symptoms of cinchonism or chronic quinine poisoning and the patient will confess to most of them. Let us take, for instance, "The Materia Medica and Therapeutics", by Mitchell Bruce, published here in Chicago. He says:

"The obvious phenomena produced by a full dose (15 to 30gr) of quinine are not by any means its most important effects. It acts most strikingly upon the nervous centres, and causes confusion of mental faculties, noises in the ears and deafness, disorders of vision (colour blindness), headache, giddiness, vomiting, and possibly prostration from involvement of the cord and circulation.

Quinine appears to reduce the amount of nitrogenous excretions, of urea and uric acid, and probably also of carbonic acid, as determined both in healthy and fevered animals, and in man. These two sets of effects, taken together, point to a powerful action of quinine in reducing the metabolism of the body, of which heat and excretions are the two most measurable products." (note)

(Author's note: This confirms my claim that all antipyretics and antiseptics are protoplasmic poisons.)

"We may, therefore, conclude that the effect of quinine in the body is to check metabolism by interfering with the odixation of protoplasm generally, with oxygenation, and with the associated actions of ferments. Thus the fall of temperature produced by quinine is due to the diminished production of heat in the body, and not to increased loss of heat."

Fever heat contracts the surface capillaries, tightly closes the skin and its organs, and thus prevents heat radiation. Therefore we have in fevers a dry, hot surface. The drug, by "reducing the metabolism", which means partial paralysis of the vital functions, suppresses the heat which is burning up the morbid matter in the system. The cold wet packs and cold ablutions do not interfere with inner heat production. They cool and relax the skin, its pores and capillaries, thereby facilitating heat radiation and the elimination of impurities from the blood. The following quotations from "Essentials of Materia Medica and Therapeutics", by H. Norris, M.D., are very significant, revealing in every paragraph the law of double effect in the immediate and remote effects of quinine in the human organism. It must be remembered that all drugs taken in small doses tend to accumulate in the system and concentrate in certain parts for which they exhibit a special affinity and then constantly exert the influences of large doses. The notes in parentheses in the following paragraphs are by myself.

"Locally, cinchona and its alkaloids are irritant and antiseptic, destroying minute organisms or inhibiting their movements.

"Internally it acts on the alimentary canal as a simple bitter, in small doses increasing the appetite and digestion; if long continued, producing indigestion and catarrh." (Note the double effect. In ordinary doses cinchona constipates. In large doses cinchona or its alkaloids irritate the mucous membrane and cause vomiting and diarrhoea followed by chronic constipation.)

"Nutrition is stimulated and the excretion of waste products increased by small doses; large doses, however, diminish the amount of urea and uric acid and phosphoric acids in the urine. In malarial fever the products of waste tissue are much decreased." (Thus interfering with elimination.)

"In the blood it interferes with the oxygen carrying function of the red corpuscles, and diminishes their number, inhibits the movements and prevent the migration of the white corpuscles, both in health and disease." (If the allopath believes in the theory of phagocytosis, why prevent the migration of the leucocytes?)

"Circulation: in small doses the cardiac action is increased; large doses, by acting on the cardiac motor ganglia, depress the heart, sometimes causing it to intermit, and finally arrest it in diastole; the blood pressure is lowered." (This means death.)

"The temperature in health is very slightly influenced, if at all; in fevers a rapid decline takes place, due to the depressive action on the blood and circulation.

"Nervous system: small doses stimulate the cerebral functions, large doses cause cinchonism, i.e., a constricted feeling in the forehead, giddiness and tinnitus aurium (ringing in the ears), with impairment of hearing and sometimes of vision; after toxic doses these symptoms are aggravated and delirium, weak pulse, coma, sometimes convulsions, and in rare cases death, supervene. It probably reduces the reflex excitability of the spinal cord.

"Cutaneous eruptions, as erythema, urticaria or herpes, are produced in some subjects by even small doses of cinchona or its alkaloids." (These eruptions appear when the drug is eliminated under natural methods, in healing crises.)

From these various quotations it plainly appears that quinine is an antiseptic, germ killer and anti-fever remedy because it is a protoplasmic poison; it benumbs, paralyses and kills red corpuscles, depresses the heart and respiratory centres, and in brief, reduces fever symptoms because it retards all vital functions. It "cures" catarrh because it acts as an astringent on the mucous membranes — that is, it contracts and paralyzes the cells and glandular structures of these membranes so that they cannot throw off the morbid matter which nature is trying to eliminate. Medical students in our colleges are constantly warned not to give quinine in large quantities or continued doses to railroad men, because it may cause colour blindness and deafness. They are told that this might cause a misunderstanding of colour signals and thereby produce railroad accidents. Whether or not other people become colour blind and deaf does not seem to be a matter of importance.

Not long ago there appeared before our public clinic a woman about forty years of age who asked for a diagnosis from the eye. Both eyes were yellow with the typical quinine colour (see Colour plate, Fig.c) and the regions of throat, lungs and bronchi displayed the dark signs of chronic and destructive catarrhal conditions. We told her at once, without a word of information from her, that she was thoroughly poisoned by quinine and that in consequence she was suffering from bad chronic catarrhal conditions, bordering on tuberculosis. "Yes," she said, "I have been coughing and expectorating for a year and the doctors tell me that I have consumption. Two years ago I was a perfectly well woman and strong as a man. My husband died with consumption and I, after reading some medical books, began to fear that he had infected me with the disease. The books told me that quinine was a good preventive against catarrhs, coughs and tuberculosis. Although there was nothing the matter with me at the time, I took large doses of it without a doctor's prescription, and kept on taking it until one day I dropped, senseless, on the floor. A doctor was called and after hearing my story told me I had taken too much quinine; that I was suffering from the chronic after effects of the drug. I then began to cough and have grown worse ever since." In this case, without doubt, the drug which was taken to prevent the disease produced it in most terrible reality.

The perfection of the microscope and the discovery of microorganisms of disease gave a new and great impetus to allopathic science. In the germ theory of disease was found the solution of all therapeutic riddles, proof positive of the fallacy of the teachings of Hahnemann and a perfect justification of allopathic symptomatic and surgical treatment of disease. One of the favourite bits of evidence always produced in favour of these theories is the specific action of quinine in malarial diseases. "The Plasmodium Malariae is found in the blood of malarial patients, quinine kills the Plasmodium and the fever symptoms abate (temporarily); therefore is the Plasmodium the cause of the malaria and quinine the cure for it." In like manner, other specific germs are supposed to be the causes of the diseases after which they are named; hence the formula, "Find chemicals or serums to kill the bacteria, and cure the disease."

Let us see if this reasoning is true in the case of malaria and quinine. The allopathic theory is supported by the fact that almost all northerners who go to certain hot and moist lowland districts in tropical countries are affected by this and other tropical fevers. This seems to be sufficient proof that the cause of the disease lies entirely in certain parasitic germs, peculiar to these districts, and in the presence of mosquitoes which convey these germs into human blood. The diagnosis from the eye, as repeatedly stated, reveals the fact that the majority of human beings are more or less affected and encumbered with inherited and acquired disease taints and morbid matter. These chronic encumbrances are more pronounced in the inhabitants of colder zones, because the colder temperature retards acute elimination and because the greater consumption of meat, pork, coffee, tea and liquors, and the almost entire absence of eliminating fruits from the daily dietary, favours the accumulation of waste and morbid matter, which forms a luxuriant soil for all sorts of disease germs. When such persons arrive in the hot, moist, malarial lowlands of tropical climates, the malarial parasites and other disease germs find congenial soil in the morbid matter of their systems and produce the peculiar fermentative processes of yellow fever, cholera, malaria, etc. That these germs grow and thrive in morbid blood only, has been proved by hundreds of European vegetarians who have emigrated to tropical countries. They live in localities known as the worst fever districts in the world, in perfect immunity from tropical disorders, whilst their meat-eating, liquor- and coffee-drinking, tobacco-smoking and quinine-eating countrymen fall an easy prey to all tropical diseases and usually within a few years return to Europe ruined in health physically and mentally.

Viewpoint of Natural Therapeutics Verified by an Allopathic Teaher.

When I was a student in medical college Dr. C. was one of our professors of Materia Medica. He was an old experienced physician and in theory and practice a thorough allopath, but he had never employed quinine in the treatment of malaria. How he learned to prevent and cure this disease without drugs was one of his favourite stories. "In my younger days," he said, "before I took up the study of medicine, I travelled with a government exploring expedition through some of the worst malarial districts of Old Mexico and South America. One day I befriended a native and in return for some kindness I had shown him, he taught me how to avoid the malaria and other tropical fevers. He told me to keep my bowels open by avoiding meat and by eating plenty of fruit, and to guard against chilling at night by keeping myself well covered with woollen blankets. I followed his advice, ate plenty of fruit, kept myself well covered, so that all through the night my body was in a state of semi-perspiration, and I never contracted the fever or took a single dose of quinine. My companions would lie naked in the heated part of the tropical night, fall asleep and expose their bodies to the early morning chills. This suppressed the excretions of the skin and brought on the ague." His experience certainly proved that the malarial parasites grow in morbid blood only. As long as he kept skin and bowels active, the germs found nothing to feed on. He always added that since he began the practice of medicine, many of his patients had prevented and cured malaria by following the same simple directions. After telling his story, however, the same doctor would turn around and give a baby, two years old, a dose of quinine for a simple cold.

A medical student who heard me repeat this story tried to explain the doctor's experience as follows: "The particular kind of mosquito which carries the malaria germ is active only during the night. Keeping his body covered while asleep prevented infection." This argument does not hold good, because the little pests are awake and busy during the evening hours and in the early morning as well as during the night.

Neurasthenia Caused by Quinine.

Some years ago I happened to attend a clinic in a neighbouring college. One of the patients was a young man about thirty
years of age, a cigar maker by trade. Examination brought out
an imposing array of nervous symptoms. The unanimous ver-
dict of the assembled doctors and students was "neurasthenia". The professor in charge of the clinic asked for a
definition of "neurasthenia". Having listened to a long recital
of nervous and mental symptoms he said, "In my last paper
before the County Medical Association I described this mysterious modern nervous derangement as follows: 'A patient
suffers from a multitude of nervous symptoms; headaches,
backaches, neuro-muscular weakness, the feeling of weight
on the brain, mental irritability, ringing in the ears, insomnia,
etc.' You cannot find any local or constitutional diseases to
account for the nervous symptoms; in fact you do not know
what ails the patient — that is neurasthenia."

In the meantime I, myself, examined the eyes of our subject and the professor asked me for my diagnosis of the case. I
gave it as my opinion that the man was suffering from chronic
cinchonism, or quinine poisoning. Asked what made me
think so, I replied that the iris showed very prominently the
yellow colour of quinine in the regions of stomach, intestines,
liver and spleen. The two last organs also showed signs of
inflammation and enlargement, which usually go with
chronic quinine poisoning. To corroborate the diagnosis I
asked the patient if he had suffered from malaria. "Oh yes,"
he answered. "I lived in the South and suffered from malaria
for four years, and had to come north on account of it." "Did
you take much quinine?" "Yes, almost daily for four years." I
then asked him for other symptoms of chronic cinchonism as
given in standard materia medica; he admitted that he suffered from practically all of them. Having finished my
examination, I remarked to the professor that the history of
the patient, as well as his symptoms, seemed to justify my
diagnosis. The professor dismissed the subject with the curt
reply: "That was orthodox treatment; it has nothing to do with
our diagnosis."

It may seem harsh to "tell tales out of school", but this
happened in open clinic, within hearing of the patient. What

about hundreds and thousands of other patients who suffer all
their lives on account of that sort of diagnosis and treatment.

Paresis Caused by Quinine.

Three years ago a lady brought her husband to us for
examination. His mind was in a weakened condition so that
he could not act for himself. The best physicians in her home
city in Wisconsin, and two of the great nerve specialists in
Chicago had examined the patient and told her that his mental
breakdown was caused by overwork. The Chicago "specialists" had charged her fifty dollars apiece for looking at him
and making this profound diagnosis. Nowadays "the strenuous life" is made the scapegoat for a good many troubles that
are beyond the ken of the "expert" and "specialist". On
examining the iris I found the yellow colour of quinine in the
areas of brain, liver and spleen; also to some extent in the
stomach and bowels, indicating heavy quinine poisoning.
When I informed the lady that her husband was suffering
from chronic quinine poisoning, she answered, "This may be
possible, because during the last few years he has taken
quinine almost daily to cure his hay fever. A doctor gave him
a quinine prescription for this purpose and after that he kept
on taking it of his own accord." This left no doubt about the
correctness of the records in the iris.

The case proved to be beyond redemption. Before death
liberated him from his earthly suffering he had to pass for a
year through the revolting conditions which characterize the
gradual breaking down of the brain tissue, labelled "paresis"
by the medical profession. This man came from an exceptionally healthy family. He himself had never been sick in his
life until he began to suffer from hay fever. His habits of living had been very temperate and he was known as one of the
best all-round college athletes in his state. Surely the work of
a cashier in a small town was not sufficient to cause physical
and mental breakdown in a man of that type.

Quinine.
Allopathic Uses.

1. Appetizer and bitter tonic during convalescence,
general debility, and while taking depressing remedies
like mercury, lead, etc.

2. Against all febrile diseases, especially malaria and all conditions resulting from it. "Of unquestionable value if freely administered".

3. Against splenic leukaemia.

4. Local anaesthetic, injected with urea hydrochloride for minor surgical operations — used instead of cocaine.

5. Rectal injection against amoebic dysentry.

6. Against painful nervous conditions. "Shows well marked effects, acting as cardiac and central nervous depressant".

7. Menstrual stimulant and abortive.

Accidental Poisoning.

Malarial preventatives.

Patent tonics. Hair tonics.

Toxicology:

"Converted in the stomach into quinine hydrochloride, a readily diffusable salt which enters the blood stream within a few minutes after ingestion. Decreases functional activity of all forms of protoplasm. Reduces number of leucocytes (Hence its suppressive action on inflammatory processes). Binds oxygen more firmly to haemoglobin thus interfering with proper oxygenation and decreasing the nitrogenous output". Clearly therefore, quinine reduces temperature by suppressing the production and not by facilitating the liberation of heat.

The most important symptoms of Cinchonism (chronic quinine poisoning) are the following:

1. Congested frontal headaches.

2. Sensation of fullness or pressure at top of head.

3. Ringing in ears.

4. Disturbances of vision (dilation of pupils with imperfect response to accommodative effect). Colour-blindness.

5. Gastro-intestinal and renal irritation often accompanied by haemoglobinuria.

6. Itchy skin eruptions.

7. Restless, unrefreshing sleep, dizziness, drowsiness and debility.

8. Nervousness, neurasthenia and insanity. Note the

similarity between cinchonism and neurasthenia.

Elimination of Drug in Healing Crises.

1. Through the skin causing itchy eruptions resembling scarlatina or measles.

2. Through the kidneys as amorphous alkaloid which irritates urinary passages, often causing haematuria.

3. Elimination of drug in healing crises frequently accompanied by taste of the drug in the mouth.

4. Through acute catarrhal elimination, purging and haemorrhoidal discharges.

Signs in Iris.

The drug shows most prominently in the brain region in yellow pigments ranging from whitish to reddish tints; variation probably due to chemical admixtures. In severe poisoning the yellowish discolourations show also in stomach, intestines, liver and spleen, in the latter organs especially in cases of chronic malaria (Colour plate, Fig.c)

CHAPTER XIV
IODINE
(Colour Plate, Figs.b and c)

The most prominent alterative next to mercury is iodine. Judging from the records in the iris, it must be one of the most popular drugs used by the regular school of medicine, for we find iodine spots in the eyes of about one fourth of all the subjects we examine. No other poisonous drug shows more plainly in the iris, but the signs vary according to the mode of absorption. If taken internally, the poison shows in the iris as bright red, reddish brown, pink or orange coloured spots or blotches (Colour plate, b and c). These spots are frequently transparent so that the underlying tissues of the iris can be discovered. Sometimes they are surrounded by white borders indicating that the poison is causing irritation and inflammation or that it is in the process of elimination in a healing crisis.

Where the iodine has been applied externally and has been absorbed through the skin, the signs in the iris are of a pinkish hue and appear in the form of streaks, broom-like markings or reddish clouds. It is understood that these signs are visible in the areas of the iris corresponding to those parts of the body in which the poison has accumulated. The signs of iodine which has been taken internally are often similar to itch spots, still with a little practice they can be distinguished readily enough. The iodine spots are usually of a brighter red and more diffuse than the itch or psora spots. Sometimes the history of the patient also helps to clear up the doubt. While other drugs exhibit a well defined affinity for certain portions of the body, we find iodine spots almost everywhere, frequently in the areas of liver, kidneys, stomach and bowels, lungs, pancreas and the brain.

Iodine as Described in Allopathic Materia Medica.
Iodine (Iodum) is a solid non-metallic element. It is obtained from native iodides and iodads and from the ashes of sea weeds. Its principal preparations are potassium iodide, sodium iodide, the tincture of iodine, iodine liniment and iodine ointment. Its actions and uses are thus described in "Materia Medica and Therapeutics", by J. Mitchell Bruce, used as a text book in leading allopathic medical colleges in England and America.

"Externally applied, iodine is a powerful irritant and vesicant, decomposing organic molecules, and entering into loose chemical combination with the albuminous constituents of the parts. At the same time it stains the epidermis a deep brown; causes considerable pain; and is absorbed into the blood, partly by the skin and partly by the air of respiration in the form of vapour. It is also a very powerful antiseptic and disinfectant."

This description of the action of iodine again confirms our claim that all antiseptics, antipyretics, germicides and antitoxins are powerful protoplasmic poisons and that their medicinal action depends upon their life destroying qualities.

"The tincture, strong solution, and ointment of iodine are extensively used as stimulants and disinfectants to foul callous ulcers, much like silver nitrate; as vegetable parasiticides in ringworm; and as counter irritants in subacute or chronic inflammation of joints, periostium, lymphatic glands, the pleura and the lungs, for which purpose the ointments of lead iodide and of mercuric oxide are also applied. In these instances the chief effect is doubtless stimulation —"

Iodine acts as a counter irritant and stimulant because it is a protoplasmic poison. All poisons have a stimulating and irritating effect on the tissues of the body because the organism as a whole, its organs, cells and living molecules, and the vital forces animating them, are aroused to intense activity by the effort to repel the hostile invader. Temporary benefit from irritation or stimulation is counterbalanced by the inevitable reaction and "the decomposition of organic molecules".

"But a certain amount of the iodine is absorbed, and acts specifically as will presently be described. Iodine in solution is injected into cysts, goitres, hydroceles, etc., with much success . . . ."

The specific action of iodine here referred to, consists in the "drying up" of glandular structures. This may destroy them as effectually as extirpation with the surgeon's knife. I fail to understand how this can be called "a cure". Later I shall give some instances of the chronic after effects of such "absorbent" treatment.

"Compounds of iodine with creosote and various soothing volatile substances, such as chloroform and ether, are used as continuous inhalations in the so-called "antiseptic" treatment of phthisis, bronchitis and other forms of chronic pulmonary disease."

It is hard to tell whether these antiseptics will more quickly and effectually destroy the lung tissue or the disease germs. (See first quotation.)

"In the stomach and bowels, although it is gradually converted into sodium iodide, the irritant effects of free iodine are continued, with abdominal pain and diarrhoea as the result . . . . In the blood the element is at first found combined with sodium; but the salt appears to be decomposed and the iodine for a time set free, for some of the red corpuscles are broken down (if the amount of iodine is large), and bloody effusions and bloody urine make their appearance. Such results are to be carefully avoided in practice. . . ."

This, too, indicates the destructive effect of the drug.

Specific Actions and Uses.

"The lymphatic glands are reduced in size by iodine, which is extensively used for scrofulous and other chronic enlargements of the glands, whether applied locally as iodine, or administered internally as the iodides."

The cause of this is explained above.

"The excretion of iodine by the mucous membrane of the respiratory tract is of most interest to the therapist. In certain subjects and probably when potassium iodide contains free iodine as an impurity, its exhibition produces a series of unpleasant symptoms known as 'iodism', consisting of coryza, the watery discharge from the nose being sometimes profuse; sneezing; severe pain of a bursting character over the frontal sinuses, commonly called 'headache'; swelling and redness of the gums, hard palate and fauces; foulness of the tongue, and increase of the mucus of the mouth; cough and frothy expectoration and a sense of heat and rawness in the trachea and chest. . . .

"In escaping by the skin the liberated iodine produces in certain individuals peculiar eruptions; papular, acneform, vascular or pustular, rarely purpuric . . . . Potassium iodide is said to be an antigalactogogue (milk suppressant).

The symptoms just described frequently manifest during the elimination of the drug in healing crises. The worst effects, because deep seated and obscure, are not mentioned. Here I may briefly state that in many cases we have found iodine to give rise to Bright's disease, diabetes, paresis, ulcers of the stomach and bowels, chronic diseases of pancreas, spleen and lungs. Some specific cases I shall describe later on.

Does Iodine Eliminate Mercury?

"Certain poisons which have intimately associated themselves with the albuminous structures, are disengaged from these combinations by iodine. Lead and mercury may be swept out of the tissues with the assistance of potassium iodide, administered for plumbism and hydrargyrism respectively.

"The principal application, however, of iodine is the treatment of syphilis. Either the virus of this disease is thus eliminated from the system, or iodine hastens the life and disappearance of the small-celled growth by which syphilis is characterized. It is especialy valuable in the tertiary forms of syphilis, when mercury cannot always be given with advantage; and nodes and other superficial enlargements, gummata in the viscera, and certain forms of skin disease may be very successfully treated with the potassium salt. The same precautions must be observed with respect to the general health, and especially the preservation of digestion, in the case of iodine, as are laid down under the head of mercury."

Various preparations of iodine are administered to couteract the effects of mercury, which are usually labelled tertiary syphilis. Old school materia medica assumes that iodine neutralizes and eliminates the mercury. When the latter has been taken to the point of saturation and exudes from the body through ulcers, abscesses, haemorrhoids, etc., iodine arrests the acute activity aroused by the mercury and paralyzes nature's effort to throw it off. Both poisons recede into the organism and continue their work of destruction. That this is true is proved by the signs of the poisons in the iris and the accompanying symptoms in the organs affected. It is again Beelzebub against the devil. The so called tertiary syphilitic usually suffers as much from iodine poisoning as from mercury. It counteracts the mercurial sores and ulcerations because it is a protoplasmic poison. It "dries up" and "absorbs" healthy tissues as well as diseased ones.

Dr. A. Farrington (a homoeopath) says, in his Clinical Materia Medica, when speaking of the destructive after effects of iodine:

"Iodine is an absorbent; it has the property of causing absorption, particularly of glandular tissues, involving, finally, even nervous structures. We find, for instance, in persons who are poisoned with iodine, great emaciation. With the female, the mammary glands become atrophied and the ovaries, too, no doubt. With the male, the testicles suffer inevitable progressive loss of sexual power. The skin becomes dark yellow and tawny, dry from deficient action, the sclerotica (of the eyes) become yellow, yellow spots appear on the face and also on the body. There is excessive appetite; he is anxious and faint if he does not get his food. He is relieved while eating and yet he emaciates despite the amount of food he eats. Sooner or later the nervous system becomes involved and he is afflicted with tremor. He becomes nervous and excitable; every little annoyance which would be unnoticed in his normal condition causes trembling. He has a longing for the open air, as if the cold, fresh air gave him more breath. This gives a fair idea of the condition to which the patient is reduced by the overuse of iodine."

A lady was sent to us by a physician for diagnosis. After looking into her eyes, I at once laid my hand on her right temple and said, "There is serious trouble here; you must suffer from chronic headaches." This she at once admitted, saying, "It is that which brought me here. No one has been able to detect the cause of the trouble. Since you have discovered the locality, can you also tell me the cause?" "Certainly," I replied. "It is iodine, applied externally and absorbed through the skin. The left frontal brain area in the iris displays a large reddish streak. Do you remember when and for what the iodine was applied?" After some effort she remembered that when she was about six years old, her neck had been repeatedly painted with iodine for "swollen glands". On further enquiry she admitted that soon afterwards the headaches made their appearance and had never left her, as far as she knew, for a single waking hour. In order to "cure" the headache, she took quantities of bromides, coal tar preparations and other brain and nerve paralyzers which, of course, aggravated and complicated her chronic ailments.

My Own Experience with Iodine.

Iodine was the cause of my undertaking the study and general practice of Natural Therapeutics. About twenty years ago I was in very poor health. After giving up all hope of being cured by drugs, I went to Europe seeking relief in Nature Cure sanitariums. I was greatly surprised when one of the physicians in charge, after looking at my eyes, immediately told me the cause of all my troubles. He said, "Your right kidney and liver are ruined by iodine". I remembered that our family physician had swabbed my throat internally with iodine and painted it externally when I was a lad, twelve years old. But I never suspected that those long forgotten applications of this drug could have anything to do with the tendency to diabetes.

In my case the elimination of these and other poisons took the form of furuncles. There were at one time over twenty on my body. I allowed them to run their course without being lanced or treated with antiseptics. This proved to be the great healing crisis in my case for, after that vigorous housecleaning, I felt like one new-born. I seemed to be in perfect health and since that time have not been sick in bed for one day. Most of the spots disappeared, but some are still faintly visible as shown in Fig.16.

A patient asked me if I could explain why she had an abundance of milk for her first baby while she was unable to nurse any of the three following. I examined the iris and found in the region of the right chest and breast a broad yellowish-red streak of iodine. There were also closed lesions in the pleura and the lower lobe of the lung. I said to her, "After the birth of your first child and before the next was born you had a severe attack of pneumonia and pleurisy and your breast was painted with iodine". This she confirmed. When her first child was sixteen months old she contracted pneumonia and pleurisy and the entire right side was heavily painted with iodine. Undoubtedly, the drug had been absorbed and had dried up the mammary glands. This accounted for her inability to nurse the other childen. In several cases I have traced sexual impotence to the action of iodine on the sex organs.

Iodine.

Allopathic Uses.

1. Antiseptic dressing for wounds.

2. Stimulant and disinfectant on foul ulcers.

3. Injected into cysts, goitres, hydroceles, etc., "with much success".

4. Counter irritant in chronic inflammation of joints, periosteum, pleura, lungs and tubercular lymph nodes.

5. Metabolic stimulant for disintegrating and eliminating drugs such as mercury, lead, etc., which have intimately combined with the albuminous constituents of the body.

6. Stimulating expectorant in bronchial catarrh and pneumonia if consolidation threatens to persist.

7. Antispasmodic in asthma and emphysema.

8. Antigalactagogue. Dries up mammary glands.

9. For aneurisms as K.I. (potassium lowers blood pressure while iodine stimulates metabolism and coagulates the tissues.)

10. Used chiefly against tertiary syphilis — either causes the elimination of the spircheta or hastens the life and disappearance of the small-celled growth characterizing the disease.

Accidental Poisoning.

Workmen handling iodine. Patent goitre cures. (The world annually produces 11,000 tons of iodine for medicinal purposes. Is it any wonder that we find it so frequently in the iris?

Toxicology.

Iodine is freely absorbed into the circulation where is it resolves the red corpuscles. It rapidly passes to all tissues especially the excretory organs and lymph nodes.

Symptoms of Iodism.

1. Inflamed gums, palates and fauces.

2. Coryza with bursting pain over frontal sinuses.

3. Cough and frothy expectoration.

4. Acneform eruptions.

5. Abdominal pain, nausea, diarrhoea.

6. Glandular atrophy, especially testes, ovaries and mammae.

7. Anaemia, emaciation, and general debility.

Elimination of Drug in Healing Crises.

Catarrhal discharges from nose, sneezing, severe pain over the frontal sinuses; intense headaches; swelling and redness of the gums, hard and soft palates; foulness of the tongue; increase of mucus in the mouth; cough and frothy expectorations; papular, acneform, vascular or pustular eruptions; open sores, haemorrhoidal discharges and other symptoms according to the location of the poison in the system.

Signs in the Iris.

Described at the beginning of the chapter.

CHAPTER XV

LEAD
(Colour Plate, Fig. b)

The drug shows in the iris in the form of lead blue or bluish grey discolouration in the region of stomach and bowels. I have found the dark blue or bluish grey sign of lead many times in the eyes of painters, printers, plumbers and other workers in lead, suffering from lead poisoning or lead colic. The sign in the iris indicates that the drug has a strong affinity for the stomach, but it also affects the nerves in the upper region of the spinal cord, causing the symptoms of wrist-drop and shaking palsy or paralysis agitans. (Mercury shows a stronger affinity for the lower sections of the spinal cord, more frequently giving rise to the symptoms of locomotor ataxia.) One of the plainest diagnostic symptoms of lead poison is a blue line along the edge of the gums. I have met with many cases of lead poisoning caused through drug taking or accidental absorption of the metal.

Several years ago a patient came to me for consultation who suffered intensely from ulcers of the stomach. The eyes revealed plainly the sign of lead in the stomach area. I was unable to locate the source of the lead poisoning until I learned from the patient that for several years he had been employed in a carriage factory and that his work consisted in scraping old varnish and paint from vehicles. In this way he had inhaled and swallowed large quantities of the metal contained in the paint scrapings. Under natural treatment he made a perfect recovery. Another patient who had suffered for years with severe indigestion, neuralgia and "rheumatic pains" also showed plainly the lead sign in the region of the stomach. In this case it developed that the patient several years before had worked on the ore wharves in Cleveland, Ohio. He had been in the habit of drinking water from a spring which trickled out from under a large pile of metal bearing rocks. He became violently ill, and was taken to a hospital where the doctors diagnosed his case as metallic poisoning. While he recovered from the acute attack, he was never well afterward and was treated for several years for indigestion, muscular rheumatism and neuralgia. The eyes revealed the true nature of his acute and chronic ailments. He also made a perfect recovery under natural treatment.

Lead and mercury produce the most stubborn forms of chronic constipation. The intestinal tract in the iris of such patients frequently has a black appearance (Colour plate, e and f). Many such cases we have had to treat for six months or longer before the first white lines appeared in the black area of the stomach and intestines indicating the return to life into the paralyzed organs.

Lead.

Allopathic Uses.
1. Externally as astringent and sedative in bruises, itches, ulcers and inflamed surfaces in general.
2. As injection against chronic inflammatory discharges from vagina, urethra, ear, etc.
3. Sprains (lead water and opium).
4. Haemostat for internal haemorrhage.
5. Powerful ecbolic (producing abortion).

Accidental Poisoning.
1. Workmen handling lead, type, paint, tinfoil, etc.
2. Lead water pipes.
3. Action of acid preservers on solder in canned goods.
4. Lead coated pottery.
5. Candy and cake colours (chromate).
6. Hair dyes (sulphide).
7. Glasswear.

Toxicology.
Enters through skin, respiratory and alimentary tracts.

Circulates as albuminate of lead, reducing red corpuscles and salts. Is soon taken up by tissues and obstinately retained.

Symptoms of Plumbism.

1. Blue line along the edge of gums.

2. Malnutrition.

3. Profound anaemia. Icterus Saturius.

4. Lead colic. Stubborn constipation.

5. Neuromuscular pain and rigidity often mistaken for rheumatism.

6. Paralysis saturia (lead palsy, wrist-drop, ankle-drop). Symmetrical, starting as feebleness and stiffness. Paralysis agitans.

7. Retinitis secondary to arterisclerosis and interstitial nephritis. Vertigo and delirium in severe cases.

Elimination of the Drug in Healing Crises:

Severe gastritis, haemorrhages from stomach, haemorrhoidal discharges; skin eruptions and ulcers (similar to mercury), sores in the mouth; bleeding of gums; severe nervous symptoms.

Signs in Iris.

See the introductory paragraph in this chapter.

CHAPTER XVI

ARSENIC
(Colour plate, Fig.b)

Several cases of accidental arsenical poisoning have already been cited earlier in this volume. Another similar case was that of a farmer who came to us suffering from great enlargement of the spleen and from pernicious leukaemia. His eyes showed the signs of arsenic very plainly, but for several weeks we were unable to trace the source of the poisoning, until I mentioned paris green. He then told me that for many years he had sprayed his potato vines with a preparation containing large amounts of paris green. He remembered that frequently the wind had driven the spray into his face. This solved the mystery. He came too late, however, and succumbed to the effects of the arsenical poisoning.

Several years ago it was discovered that arsenical poisoning was frequently due to the inhalation of poisonous emanations from wall paper that owed its green colour to paris green. Since then the use of paris green in the manufacture of wall paper has been prohibited by law. If arsenical poisoning can occur by inhaling the poisonous emanation from wall paper, what about taking arsenic in large quantities in Fowler's solution, salvarsan and other medical preparations? While the first effect of the drug seems to be tonic and stimulating, this is soon followed by greater weakness and collapse. A well known trick of dishonest horse dealers consists in giving more or less decrepit horses large doses of arsenic. This acts as a powerful stimulant on the animal. His coat becomes glossy, the eyes sparkle with the fire of youth and he prances about in high spirits. But the unwary purchaser finds to his astonishment within a few days that the animal has lost its youthful vigour and fine appearance.

The effect of the poison on human beings suffering from anaemia is not one whit better. Whenever the drug is discontinued, the anaemic symptoms reappear in worse form than before. Many people contract a habit for the drug which is very difficult to overcome.

Some of the worst cases of chronic multiple or peripheral neuritis that have come under my observation were caused by prolonged medication with arsenical preparations. The notorious salvarsan is a powerful preparation of arsenicum. The formula is $C_{12}H_{12}O_2N_2As_2$. This concoction has never cured a single case of blood poisoning. At the best it has only temporarily suppressed symptoms. Many patients have come under our care and treatment who were entirely ruined by it. A year ago we had under our care two cases who were made blind by its use. One of these patients had enjoyed good eyesight until he received four salvarsan injections. After each treatment his eyesight became weaker. After the fourth he could only dimly distinguish objects. Too late it dawned upon him that the salvarsan was destroying his eyesight. The other patient had a similar experience. Her eyesight greatly improved under natural treatment. The man, a Bohemian saloon-keeper, had not the necessary intelligence to understand Nature Cure, and went back to poison treatment. I do not know what became of him, but I am certain that he has not regained his eyesight. Another case treated with salvarsan in one of the large Chicago hospitals, went insane. The doctors in charge of the case said it was paresis, due to syphilis in early life. They pronounced the case incurable and sent him to the State Asylum for the Insane at Elgin. Later his friends consulted me about the case and on my advice had him paroled and brought to our institution for treatment. He improved rapidly, as the "606" was eliminated from his system, and three months after coming to us he failed to return from his daily walk. One of our attendants went to his house to see if he was there and found him working at his jeweler's bench. He has never had a relapse since. I could relate dozens of instances where the "606" worked similar havoc in different ways, but space does not permit. On the other hand I

have never come across a single case of so called chronic
blood poisoning that has been permanently cured by this concoction. It was sprung on humanity and immediately accepted by the medical profession and the laity in all civilized
countries simply on account of the reputation of Dr. Ehrlich
as a great light in science. On November 21st, 1917, the
following news item appeated in the Chicago Daily Tribune:

"Doctors Cheer at Discovery of New Cures"

"Announcement of two discoveries of world wide
importance in the cure of tetanus and syphilis were made
today at the annual fall meeting of the National
Academy of Science, held at the university of Pennsyl-
vania. Discovery of the new drug, known as A-189, was
made at the Rockefeller Institute after experiments dat-
ing from the outbreak of the world war. It means virtually the medical independence of America from
Germany. The new drug, an organic arsenical compound, can be prepared in this country at a nominal cost
of five cents a dose wholesale, whereas the wholesale
price of salvarsan is now $3.50 a dose.

But the most important feature of the new invention is
the fact that it develops greater resistance for the
spirochaetal infections without doing as much damage
to the cells of the body."

In the last paragraph of this report it is admitted that the
old preparation of salvarsan did much to damage the system.
New preparations of old poisons are usually introduced to the
profession with similar phrases, i.e., "The old preparations of
this drug were known to have very serious side effects upon
the system, but this new product of our laboratories produces
all the good effects of the drug without any of its destructive
after effects." This kind of announcement holds good until a
new preparation is discovered.

Allopathic Uses.

1. Externally as caustic (with iodine) against lupus,
keratosis and new growth of skin (does not act until
absorbed).
2. Internally against chronic skin eruptions (with
sulphur).

3. Lues as salvarsan (606) neosalvarsan (914) and sodium cacodylate.

4. Hay fever and asthma.

5. Popular tonic haematinic used with iron for leukaemia, pernicious anaemia, and symptomatic anaemia resulting from tuberculosis, malaria, gout, rheumatism, etc.

6. General tonic and alterative in all cases of perverted metabolism. "5 gtt. Fowler's Solution t.i.d. Increase 1 gtt. daily until eyelids become oedamatous or until faint darting pains are felt in abdomen. Reduce dose and continue until the above symptoms reappear. Reduce again and repeat."

Accidental Poisoning.

1. Paris green, "Rough on Rats", napthalein and other insect and vermin exterminators.

2. Cloth dyes. Wool in manufacture is treated with arsenic as a preservative. Glazes and wall papers.

3. "Cancer cures". Condition powders.

4. Taxidermists and furriers.

5. Cosmetics.

Toxicology.

Readily diffusable, producing excessive oxidation and combustion. Toxic only to organisms with a central nervous system.

Symptoms of Chronic Arsenical Poisoning.

1. Waxy complexion with loose, brittle hair and nails.

2. Arsenical eczema.

3. Puffed eyelids, conjunctival infection. Photophobia. Lachrymation.

4. Catarrhal discharges from all mucous surfaces.

5. Numbness and tingling in the extremities.

6. Cold drizzling sensation over back.

7. Neuralgia and peripheral neuritis.

8. Progressive muscular atrophy.

9. Engorgement of liver, spleen and lymphatic glands.

Elimination of Drug in Healing Crises.

1. Kidneys, bowels, liver.

2. Skin, in form of arsenical eczema, boils, running sores, dandruff and shedding of hair.

3. Catarrhal dischrges from all mucous surfaces. Retained longest in bones, ligaments and other hard tissues.

Signs in Iris.

Arsenic, the third drug in the group of alteratives, shows in the outer margin of the iris in white flakes resembling snowflakes or beaten white of egg. We find these signs in the eyes of many people who have taken the poison in medicines and tonics or who have absorbed it accidentally (Colour plate, Fig.b).

CHAPTER XVII
BROMIDES
(Colour plate, Figs a & e)

The salts of bromine most commonly used are potassium, ammonium and sodium bromide. These salts act as depressants and narcotics, particularly to the brain and nervous system. They lessen the sensitiveness of the nerves and their conductivity and are also powerful depressants on the heart and sex organs, often causing loss of sex power. Bromides show in the iris as white or yellowish white discolourations. They appear in the form of a crescent in the upper regions of the iris, indicating that the drug exhibits a special affinity for the brain and sympathetic nervous system. (Colour plate, a-e). The more strongly marked this sign in the iris the more symptoms of chronic bromism will be exhibited by the patient. A very noticeable symptom of chronic bromide poisoning is a peculiar acne-form rash. The eruptions on the face and neck may turn into abscesses and ulcers. Frequently the victims of bromism exhibit erythema and copper coloured blotches. They also suffer from digestive disturbances. Mental symptoms are prominent, there being a distinct action on the blood vessels of the brain; these blood vessels contract causing anaemia and atrophy of tissues, weakening and loss of memory, defective coordination of muscular activity, difficulty in walking and tremor of limbs.

J. Mitchell Bruce, M.D., in his "Materia Medica and Therapeutics", says:

"The great vital centres of the medulla are depressed by bromides; respiration becomes weaker and slower, whence, possibly, part of the value of the drug in whooping cough. The heart also is slowed and weakened in its action — the spinal centres, nerves and muscles are all depressed by bromides, the latter so much so that the convulsions of strychnine poisoning cannot be induced".

This confirms my assertion that all sedatives, hypnotics and narcotics are merely brain and nerve paralyzers.

The salts of bromine, in addition to serving as painkillers and sleep producers, are the great epileptic remedy of the old school of medicine. It matters not where the epileptic seeks relief from his terrible malady — whether he consults the doctor on the next corner or the high priced "specialist"; whether he buys nostrums of an advertising quack or visits the great sanitariums for epileptics in Europe; the treatment is the same — bromides in some form or other. This treatment may be varied sometimes by the use of other brain paralyzing agents, such as chloral, cannabis indica, etc., but these, like the bromides, merely give temporary, fictitious relief; they never cure the disease. Professors in medical colleges freely acknowledge this to their students. The bromides are given primarily to suppress the epileptic convulsions. Unfortunately, however, they benumb and paralyze not only the centres of the brain connected with the convulsions, but the entire organ, some parts suffering more than others. This explains the gradual loss of memory, mental decline, progressive paralysis and final idiocy of the victims of bromism. These chronic complications are not due to the disease itself, but to the paralyzing effect of the drug.

Medical science has failed to discover the "epileptic centre", that is, the locality of the brain especially affected in the epileptic convulsions. The discovery was made through the diagnosis from the iris, in the following way, by the Rev. N. Liljequist, a Swedish clergyman, who has devoted his life to the study of this interesting science and who has written a most instructive book on the subject. Liljequist one day examined a man suffering from epilepsy. The disease had been caused by an accident in a saw-mill. A saw burst, a piece of it striking the man behind the left ear, burying itself deeply in the bones of the skull. The epileptic convulsions dated from that time. Evidently the condition was due to pressure on the brain, caused by the piece of steel, which had penetrated the skull. Liljequist looked into the iris for a sign of the wound in the head and found a well defined lesion in the left iris. Afterwards, when examining the eyes of epileptics he always looked for signs of disease in this area of the iris and seldom failed to discover indications of abnormal conditions in that locality.

My experience has been the same. In almost every case of epilepsy I find the signs of drug poisoning, of nerve rings, or of acute and chronic lesions in the iris area of the left cerebellum (See chart, area 3). Ten years ago Mr. L. came to me for examination. His left iris showed a marked lesion in area 3. It was apparently the sign of an injury, and when I examined the skull I found behind the left ear deep scars radiating from the depression. The location of the lesion in the iris and the scars behind the ear made me think at once of epilepsy, and I asked him whether he was not affected by the malady. He answered, "This is the trouble about which I have come to consult you; when I was four years old I had a fall and crushed in the bones of the skull behind the left ear. Immediately following the accident I went into spasms and convulsions and have suffered with epilepsy ever since". The findings in this case fully confirmed the discovery of Liljequist. It will be seen that the epileptic area lies in close proximity to the ear. Physiology teaches us that one of the functions of the internal mechanism of the ear is to aid in the maintenance of equilibrium. These centres, therefore, must be the ones affected in epileptic convulsions, for muscular coordination and the sense of equilibrium are instantly and completely inhibited in such attacks as evidenced by the sudden fall and violent spasms.

Iridology has been of incalculable value, not only in discovering the location of the epileptic centre, but also in throwing new light on the cause of the dreadful ailment. Undoubtedly, in the instance of Mr. L. whose skull was injured by a fall, the disease was caused by pressure of the indented bones, and therefore seemed to be fitting case for surgical operation. Fortunately for him he was not operated upon. I say fortunately, because trephining of the skull has proved to be anything but a blessing. For a time the operation was popular in the hospitals of Vienna, but it was found that most of these "successful" operations were, in the course of years, followed by serious brain diseases. It has been practically abandoned as a cure for epilepsy except in cases of accidental injury to the bony structure of the skull similar to the one above described. In many instances the removal of the pieces of bone pressing on the brain has undoubtedly cured cases of epilepsy, insanity and other mental disorders, but the after effects of trephining, on the whole, have not been desirable.

In many cases of this kind adhesions are formed which draw tissues out of their proper alignments and interfere with circulation and nutrition. The developments in Mr. L.'s case proved that, at least in some instances, epilepsy caused by injury to the skull can be cured by natural methods of treatment applied to the organism as a whole. When he came to us for treatment his condition was serious. The attacks displayed especial severity at night. An attendant had to be with him constantly. Aside from the typical brief spasms, he exhibited a peculiar form of convulsions, which I have not observed in any other case. For hours at a time he would be tossing about in spasms, in a dazed, semi-conscious condition. Within six months, however, the convulsions ceased entirely. He remained with us nine months longer, undergoing the regular regimen without experiencing a recurrence of the old trouble. It would seem probable that osteopathic cranial technique would be a valuable help in the natural treatment of epilepsy.

In many instances we have, by means of Iridiology, traced the exciting cause of the disorder to abnormal conditions of the digestive organs. Several cases resulted from irritation by worms, others from certain forms of indigestion. The latter patients were invariably addicted to voracious overeating. A certain form of indigestion, due to an abnormal condition of the stomach, and to overeating, affects the solar plexus, and from there the impulse to convulsions is transmitted to the epileptic brain centre. In such cases we found fasting to be of great benefit in overcoming the abnormal appetite, as well as in curing the digestive disturbance. In patients of this type we have observed that the convulsions begin with the undulatory movements in the stomach region and thence travel upwards to the brain.*

It is a fact that epilepsy often comes and goes with rheumatic conditions and no doubt many cases are due to excess of either phosphoric or uric acid in the organism. These acids are powerful stimulants and irritants of nerve and brain tissues and their activity must be held in check by sodium and sulphur. Protein foods abound in the acid producing elements, phosphorus and nitrogen, but are lacking entirely in the acid binding alkaline elements. We can readily see why a one sided meat-and-egg-white bread-potato-coffee-pie diet may produce nervous ailments, such as epilepsy, St. Vitus' dance, hysteria, nervous excitability and sexual overstimulation. Naturally the cure of such abnormal excitability of nerve and brain tissues lies in a reduction of the acid producing proteins and carbohydrates and in an increased use of fruits and vegetables, which are rich in the acid binding and eliminating organic salts.

Years ago, when my professional shingle was adorning one of the old mansions of sooty, gasoline scented Michigan Boulevard, a southern lady came to me with her son who was about twenty-two years old. His blue eyes displayed a heavy scurf rim. The dark pigmentation was especially marked in the areas of feet and legs, and it protruded like a "V" into the field of the left cerebellum. In this area were visible also segments of several nerve rings. The upper iris displayed very distinctly the whitish half-moons of bromides. The stomach and intestines exhibited the light yellowish discolouration peculiar to scrofulous elimination through these organs. (This discolouration of the intestinal field is often mistaken for the yellowish signs of quinine and sulphur). This data given, the rest was easy. I addressed the yound man as follows: "You have always suffered from poor circulation, cold, clammy, sweaty hands and feet". "Yes, that is so". "You suppressed the foot-sweat". "Yes, that is so. I was playing with a football team and perspiration of the feet troubled me very much. I used drying powders and cured it". "Soon after that you had

---

* It would seem probable that osteopathic cranical technique would be a valuable help in the natural treatment of epilepsy.

attacks of dizziness and fainting spells and then regular
epileptic fits". "Yes, that is true". "Since then you have taken
bromides in large quantities but, instead of curing the disease,
it has grown worse. Lately your memory has been very much
weakened. There is a lack of concentration and at times great
physical lassitude and mental stupour". "It is worse that
that", answered his mother; "of late he has frequently left
home for his office and landed in a different part of the city
without knowing how he came there. Once, in a dazed condition, he was nearly killed by a street car. It seems that nothing
can be done for him. I have been travelling with him now for
three years from one specialist to another, but without
avail".

"All this is very plain, Madam", I replied. "As long as
you adhere to allopathy, it matters not how many authorities
you consult, the treatment is bromides and bromides and
nothing but bromides. These so called sedatives are in reality
brain paralyzers. They are given with the idea of paralyzing
the brain centres in which the epileptic convulsions arise, but
unfortunately these agents do not confine their benumbing
influence to the left back brain, which is the seat of these disturbances. You notice that these half-moons in his eyes
extend more or less over the whole brain region. (Colour
plate, a-e). Bromism paralyzes the speech centre in one,
memory in another, the centre for "locality" in another,
according to where the poison happens to concentrate. These
signs in the eye also explain why the consumers of these
drugs are slowly but surely turned into idiots and paralytics".
"Then you think there is no hope for him", sadly interupted
his mother. "There is no hope for him, Madam", I replied, "by
the bromide route; but under natural treatment his chances of
recovery are very good indeed. Suppression of the foot-sweat
threw the scrofulous taints, in process of elimination through
the feet, into the cerebellum and this causes the periodical
irritation of the "epileptic centre". Natural methods of living
and treatment will eliminate these systemic poisons and thus
remove the cause of the trouble".

Deeply impressed by the diagnosis and by my explanation of the natural methods of treatment, she concluded to
leave the young man under our care. I then explained the law

of crises and told them to look for five or six weeks of steady
improvement, then for a temporary return of the old conditions, gastric disturbances, nose bleed, perspiration of hands
and feet, nervous depression, homesickness, etc. After the
mother's departure there arrived in due season a letter from
the father, which ran as follows: "Dear Son: Dr. X., our
family physician, after listening to your mother's report,
informs me that your doctor and his Nature Cure are a hum-
bug and a fake. I want you to return home without delay". In
reply to his Mr. B. Jr., wrote to his father: "So far I have
obeyed you in everything, but in this matter, which concerns
me so deeply, I am going to follow my own judgement. Our
family physician is entirely ignorant of this system, while
Dr.L. has studied Allopathic medicine in addition to his
Natural Therapeutics. Dr. X. does not know what he is talk-
ing about and is not competent to judge". The preliminary
improvement made in his case was marked and rapid. The
bromide eruptions and the dull, stupid expression of the face
cleared in six weeks and the patient looked the picture of
health. Convulsions had decreased from two or three daily to
about one a week. In the latter part of the sixth week the iris
area corresponding to the intestines became covered with a
white film. I informed the patient that a bowel crisis was
approaching and within twenty-four hours my prediction was
verified by the development of a lively diarrhoea. This lasted
several days and subsided without interference on our part.
At this stage I gave the patient one dose of homoeopathic sulphur in high potency. The convulsions now came thick and
fast and with great severity. One morning his pillow was
covered with blood from a nose bleed. At times his hands and
feet were dripping wet. The perspiration was of a disagreeable, sweetish odour, peculiar to these epileptic crises. At this
time he felt very much depressed, discouraged and homesick,
and if it had not been for my accurate prediction and description of almost every crisis symptom, he would have followed
his father's advice and taken the next train home. By means of
a magnifying mirror he himself saw the black patches in the
areas of the left cerebellum and feet interwoven with white
lines, indicating the active elimination of scrofulous encumbrances. For about four weeks more these acute manifesta-

tions continued and then subsided never to return. At the end
of the fifth month he left for home in perfect health.

Bromides and Loss of Identity
Frequently we read in the daily papers about people who have
wandered away from home and lost all recollection of their
identity, their home and former occupation. Some of these
patients recover, others remain permanently affected. The
majority of these cases are caused by bromides, coal tar
poisons or other brain paralyzing drugs. The only possibility
of cure in such cases lies in thorough, systematic natural
treatment.

Idiocy and Paralysis Caused by Bromides
Some of the most pitiable wrecks of humanity are to be found
among the victims of bromism. I have known young men and
women still in their teens who walked with a tottering gait
and presented the aged and withered features of people
seventy years old, feeble in body and stunted in mind, the
stare of idiocy in their eyes, typical defectives created by
bromides and other brain and nerve paralyzing drugs.

Bromine
Allopathic Uses:
  1. Externally, elementary bromine is used occasionally
as an escharotic.
  2. Internally the bromides are used as sedatives, hypnotics and antispasmodics in acute specific fevers, acute
alcoholism, mania, hysteria, infantile convulsions,
whooping cough, hypochondriasis, general nervousness, sexual overexcitement, gastro-intestinal disorders
of reflex origin, and "with great success" in epilepsy.
Toxicology:
Is rapidly absorbed from broken skin and mucous surfaces. Circulates as sodium bromide. Appears in the secretions a few minutes after ingestion, yet its total
elimination stretches over a long period of time, so that
by repeated does the patient is kept continually under its
influence. Its sedative effect is due partly to depression
of the sensory and motor nerves, but chiefly to reduced

activity of nerve centres in brain and cord. (This confirms our claims that bromides and other sedatives and hypnotics benumb and paralyze brain and nerve matter — Author.)

Symptoms of Bromism:

1. Brom-acne, so common in drugged epileptics — is in turn treated with arsenic.
2. Yellowish discolouration of skin with formation of blisters.
3. Catarrh. Salivation.
4. Headache, dizziness and general depression.
5. Impotence.
6. Diminishes reflex excitability.
7. Neuro-muscular weakness, especially of lower extremities.
8. Premature senility, paralysis, insanity, loss of self consciousness.

Elimination of Drug in Healing Crises.

1. Kidneys (mainly). Increased urination.
2. Salivary glands, mucoid accumulations in the mouth.
3. Mucous membranes, acute catarrhal elimination.
4. Skin in form of brom.acne, so familiar in drugged epileptics — in turn treated with arsenic.
5. Abnormal perspiration, nose bleed, diarrhoea.

Signs in Iris:

White crescent in region of brain and white wreath in outer margin of the iris. (Colour plate, a-e)

CHAPTER XVIII

COAL TAR PRODUCTS
(Colour plate, Figs d & f)

Signs in the Iris:

Antikamnia produces in the the upper part of the iris a greyish white veil which looks like a thin coat of white wash (Colour plate, Figs d and f). Antifebrine, antipyrine and phenacetin produce a pigmentation proceeding from the sympathetic wreath outward, in colour ranging from grey to light yelllow. Creosote and guiacol, which are used extensively as germ killers in tuberculosis and other germ diseases, produce a greyish or ashen veil over the entire iris (Colour plate, Figs a and b). In Europe the utter uselessness of these agents and their destructive effects have been fully recognised and they have been practically abandoned. In this country, however, these poisons are still widely used. The same holds true of antitoxin and tuberculin. These serums have been practically abandoned by the most advanced European physicians, while here they are rather gaining in popularity with the medical profession. Even "harmless" germs killers, if such there be, will never prove a cure for tuberculosis, because the tubercular bacillus is the product of the disease, not its cause. It grows in morbid and decayed lung tissue only. The only way to prevent the growth and multiplication of the dreaded bacilli or their microzymes is to remove from the system the morbid and scrofulous soil in which they thrive. Elimination, not "germ killing" is the cure. Every germ killer is a protoplasmic poison, and that which weakens and kills the protoplasm of bacteria and parasites also weakens and kills the protoplasm of the normal cells of the human body.

During the last thirty years coal tar preparations have become very popular as pain-killers and hypnotics. Antipyrine, antifebrin, phenacetin, antikamnia, triasol and dozens of other preparations are obtained by the distillation of coal tar. All these agents are highly poisonous and have a depressing effect on the brain, heart and respiratory centres. The use of these agents in the form of doctor's prescriptions, headache powders, nerve soothers, and hypnotics accounts for the increase in heart disease and insanity much more than does the "strenuous life". The stimulating and soothing effect of many popular drinks, such as coca cola and bromo seltzer, is due to poisonous stimulants, hypnotics or narcotics.

A few years ago Dr. Wiley, the government chemist, exhibited at the St Louis exposition a flag of the the United States which had been coloured by aniline dyes extracted from canned goods. His investigations and laboratory experiments proved that most of the foods sold in grocery stores were adulterated not only with cheap ingredients, but also with poisonous colouring materials and antiseptics, most of which were found to be coal tar preparations. In our modern artificial life people absorb poisons in many ways which they never suspect.

Insanity and Paralysis Caused by Antikamnia

Ten years ago a patient called me up on the telephone and asked me to come to her house immediately. On arriving there I was asked to examine a woman who was sitting in a chair before us. The upper part of the iris in both eyes was covered with a greyish veil looking somewhat like whitewash (Colour plate, Fig.f.). I said to Mrs A., who had summoned me, that the woman must be suffering from coal tar poisoning, probably antikamnia or creosote, and that it must be severe enough to effect her mind. Mrs A., answered that this was correct — that the patient was mentally unbalanced and also deaf and dumb. Then she explained that the woman had been doing her cleaning and laundry work, but of late had shown signs of mental aberration, and that during the last few days the condition had become acute. A doctor was called to examine the patient. His diagnosis was "insanity from worry over business matters". The friends of the patient had told him that Bessie had lost $1,400.00 by loaning it to dishonest acquaintances. From this the doctor concluded that worry over money matters was the cause of her insanity. He recommended that she be committed to an insane asylum. Mrs A., called on the people with whom Bessie had lived and while searching her room they found a number of empty antikamnia boxes. Then both Mrs A., and her landlady remembered that Bessie had been in the habit of taking medicine for her headaches and neuralgia. This explained the source of the coal tar in the iris.

With the aid of Mr A., the patient was placed under our care and treatment. For several months she was at times violently insane. Then she began to improve and after passing through the regular healing crises her mind cleared up to such an extent that in the fifth month we entrusted her with the care of our baby. Speech and hearing, however, while somewhat improved, remain to this day very defective. Ever since her recovery under the natural treatment she has been able to make her own living as a domestic servant in private families. Worry over money matters might have unbalanced her mind but surely would not have caused loss of speech and hearing. This could be caused only by some poisonous paralyzing agent. In this case also the diagnosis from the eye proved more reliable than the testimony of the expert alienist. If she had been committed to an insane asylum it would have been for life.

Coal Tar Products
Acetanilid, Antipyrin, Creosote, Phenacetin, Antikamnia, etc.

Allopathic Uses:
1. Powerful antipyretics acting within one hour.
2. General nervous sedatives, anodynes and hypnotics, "giving complete and prompt relief in nervous headache, neuralgia, ataxia pains, gout, rheumatism, dysmenorrhoea, etc".

Accidental Poisoning:
1. Patent fever remedies and headache powders.
2. Antikamnia and other proprietary anodynes.

Toxicology:

    1. Reduction of blood alkalinity and red corpuscles (This decrease in the oxygen carrying power of the blood accounts for the antipyretic action).

    2. Depression of all vital functions with a special tendency to cardiac failure (due to aniline).

Symptoms of Coal Tar Poisoning:

    1. Undue readiness to fatigue.

    2. Despondency and loss of memory.

    3. Renal irritation.

    4. Nervousness, neurasthenia, paralysis, insanity.

Elimination of Drug in Healing Crises:

    1. Excessive perspiration and erythematous eruptions.

    2. Catarrhal discharges.

    3. Excessive urination.

    4. Nervous and mental disturbances.

CHAPTER XIX

MISCELLANEOUS DRUGS

Salicylic Acid.

Signs in the Iris:

Salicylic Acid shows in the iris as a whitish grey cloud or veil, spreading unevenly over the outer margin of the iris, being more pronounced in the upper region. It resembles a whitewash and if abundant, tends to efface the peripheral border of the iris like glycerine. It is frequently associated with the sodium ring (Colour plate, Figs a and f). The drug has a corroding effect upon the membranous linings of the digestive organs. The continued use of it leaves these structures in an atrophic condition which results in malassimilation, malnutrition and defective elimination. These conditions show in the iris by a darkening and gradual browning or blackening of the areas of the stomach and intestines. People thus affected suffer from the worst forms of wasting diseases.

Allopathic Uses:

1. Antiseptic surgical dressings.
2. For softening and removing horny skin growths.
3. Perspiring feet and night sweats.
4. Gastric and intestinal fermentation and decomposition.
5. Popular antipyretic but requires larger doses than antipyrine.
6. Chronic cystitis associated with foul alkaline urine and phosphatic deposits.
7. "Specific" against inflammatory rheumatism (used in form of salicylate of sodium or lithium); of late adminis-

tered hypodermically to avoid gastro-intestinal irritation. "Administer large doses until ringing in the ears indicates physiological saturation. Discontinue till this symptom subsides, then repeat".

Accidental Poisoning:

1. Food and drink preservatives (1 percent checks enzyme action).
2. Oil of wintergreen, gaultheria and sweet birch.
3. Aspirin, novaspirin and other "cold remedies": Salol. Salophen. Salipyrine.

Toxicology:

The "specific" action of sodium salicylate against acute inflammatory rheumatism is ascribed to the following factors:

1. "It reduces the painful swelling and inflammation" (by supressing oxidation like all coal tar products).
2. "It acts as a germicide against possible rheumatism micro-organisms" (subsequently causes renal irritation).
3. "It increases the output of nitrogenous wastes such as urea, uric acid, urates, etc." (by creating new nitrogenous wastes through irritation, and not by facilitating the elimination of already existing waste acids through the neutralising action of sodium, which shows in the iris as a "sodium ring").

Symptoms of Chronic Poisoning:

In addition to the symptoms produced by the other coal tar products, salicylic acid also gives rise to:

1. Dullness of hearing. Dimness of vision.
2. Nausea. Diarrhoea alternating with constipation.

Elimination of the Drug in Healing Crises:

1. Severe indigestion — cramps in stomach and bowels, nausea and vomiting.
2. Acne-Form and pustular skin eruption.
3. Acute catarrhal elimination.

Strychnine.
(Colour plate, Fig. a)

An alkaloid prepared from nux vomica, a white crystaline, odourless powder of intensely bitter taste.

Allopathic Uses:
A cardiac and general nervine tonic.

Acute Symptoms:
Tetanic convulsions; eyeballs prominent; pupils dilated, respiration impeded, pulse feeble and rapid.

Symptoms of Chronic Strychnine poisoning:
Weakness of the heart; sluggish circulation, low blood pressure, various forms of paralysis, indigestion; spastic contraction in the pit of the stomach.

Sign in the Iris:
The sign of strychnine is very readily discerned in the iris. It shows as a white wheel of perfect proportions around the pupil in the region of the stomach, indicating that the poison has a special affinity for this organ. On closer inspection it will be seen that this wheel is made up of fine white lines or spokes radiating from the pupil.

With the strychnine sign in the iris we find associated an atonic or atrophic condition of the stomach: hypo-acidity, indigestion, fermentation and gas formation. Like all powerful stimulants, the first tonic effects of the drug on the digestive organs and the heart are followed gradually by weakness and progressive atrophy and paralysis. As a stomachic the drug is given in the form of nux vomica. It is one of the favourite heart stimulants of the old school of medicine.

Phosphorus.
(Colour plate, Fig.f)
Phosphorus shows in the iris in whitish, greyish and faded yellow flakes and clouds in the areas of stomach, intestines, brain and limbs (Colour plate, f in lungs and throat). It was used in allopathic prescriptions more extensively in former years. I have frequently found the sign of phosphorus in people who had been treated with the drug for mumps, for nervous and mental troubles and for sexual weakness. These patients suffered from severe chronic headaches, neuro-muscular pains, variously diagnosed as neuritis, multiple neuritis and chronic rheumatism. They also suffered from stubborn chronic indigestion. During the first year after absorption of the drug, the patients suffer with chronic diarrhoea, which gradually changes into chronic constipa-

tion. I have frequently seen the sign of phosphorus in the eyes of people who became poisoned with phosphorus in match factories and in chemical laboratories. Next to mercury it is the worst form of vocational poisoning.

Allopathic Uses:
1. Rickets, osteomalacia, ununited fractures.
2. Nervous disorders, like neuralgia, mania, melancholia, sexual exhaustion.
3. Chronic pulmonary diseases.
4. Some skin diseases such as psoriasis, lupus, etc.

Accidental Poisoning:
1. Workmen handling white phosphorus.
2. Vermin poisons, matches, etc.

Toxicology:
Circulates mostly in unchanged form but is partly oxidised at the expense of haemoglobin into phosphoric and phosphorous acid. Symptoms of "Lucifer Disease" are the following:
1. Ulceration of gums and necrosis of jaws starting as carious teeth.
2. General weakness due to fatty degeneration of all tissues.
3. Hectic fever, anaemia, purpura.
4. Gastro-intestinal irritation; diarrhoea; tenderness of liver.
5. Various forms of paralysis.
6. Death from general nerve exhaustion.

Elimination of Drug in Healing Crises:
1. Deep reaching ulcers, chiefly in the mouth.
2. Itchy eruptions on the skin.
3. Haemorrhage form of jaundice resembling scurvy.
4. Intestinal tract, diarrhoeas.

Turpentine.
(Colour plate, Fig.d)
It shows in the form of dense, grey clouds, mostly in the areas of the kidneys, sexual organs and bladder.

Glycerine.
Large white clouds in the areas of skin, kidneys or lungs.

They may efface the peripheral border of the iris (Colour plate, areas 18-20-28).

Ergot.

Ergot is a parasite or "smut" of rye; it was sometimes found in rye flour of poor quality. Improved grain cleaning machinery has made poisoning from this cause of rare occurrence. This poison is sometimes used by women in attempts to induce criminal abortion (Colour plate, c, areas 14-20).

Acute and Chronic Symptoms of Ergot Poisoning.
Ergotism.

The drug causes spasmodic contraction of the arteries and schlerosis of the posterior columns of the spinal cord. The early symptoms are those of digestive derangement; later symptoms are gangrene of the fingers and toes, or painful spasmodic clinching of the hands and hyperextension of the feet.

Signs in the Iris:

Rust brown spots in various parts of the body (Colour plate, fig.c, areas 14-18). A few days ago an allopathic physician who is a good friend of mine told me about a lady whom he was treating for a fibroid tumour of the womb. He remarked that he was getting good results by the administration of ergot, that it was "starving the tumour" by constricting the blood vessels and cutting off the blood supply. Since I knew that he was not open to the philosophy of Natural Thera-peutics I refrained from disputing his argument. Being a trained scientist, how could he overlook the fact that the ergot surely would not confine its constricting and starving effects to the tumour, but that it would have the same effects upon the normal tissues and organs of the body.

Opiates and Narcotics.

Every time these drugs are used they weaken, benumb and paralyze brain and nerve matter and thereby interfere with and suppress Nature's acute healing processes and produce or aggravate chronic conditions. Recovery in many critical cases is made impossible through the depressive and paralyz-ing effects of these poisons.

Opium.
(Colour plate, Figs. b,d and e)

Opium is the oldest and most widely used anodyne and hypnotic. It is prepared from the juice of the white poppy. The
drug is used in the pure form, and from it are prepared several
alkaloids of which the principal ones are morphine and
codeine. Opium shows in the iris in pure white, straight lines
radiating in the form of a star from the pupil, or from the sympathetic wreath, especially to the upper part of the iris
(Colour plate, Figs. b and e). In allopathic doses opium acts at
first as a stimulant, then as a sedative, diaphoretic (i.e. sweat-
producer), anodyne and hypnotic. It belongs to the most popular remedies of the old school of medicine. Therefore we
frequently see the sign of the drug in the iris. When taken in
sufficient quantities it creates around the pupil, in the area of
the stomach and intestines, a greyish, white star. The poison
seems to have a special and permanent affinity for the
stomach and bowels and sympathetic nervous system, and is
one of the causes of chronic constipation in children who
have been dosed with paregoric. Many cases of lifelong
chronic constipation and indigestion we have traced back to
paregoric and other baby soothers used in infancy and
early childhood.

Laudanum.

Laudanum is a tincture of opium. It contains 44 grains of
opium per ounce. It shows in the iris similarly to opium.

Paregoric.

Paregoric is a mixture of opium, camphor, glycerine, annis
seed, benzoic acid and alcohol. One half ounce of paregoric
contains one grain of opium.

Morphine.

Morphine is the principal alkaloid of opium, and its action is
similar to that of the mother drug. It is used frequently as a
sedative in heart disease, nervous disorders, asthma, coughs,
catarrhs and mental diseases. It acts more promptly when
injected subcutaneously. Helpless indeed would be the modern physician without the morphine syringe. How often must

it serve as a deceptive substitute for real relief and cure. How grateful are the patient and his friends for the prompt relief from pain. But they do not realize the destructive after effects. They do not realize that momentary relief has been bought at the expense of the fighting power of the organism and that only too often the seductive and exhalting effect of the poison makes a "dope fiend" for life.

Though morphine is closely related to opium, its signs in the iris differ somewhat from those of the latter. It creates in the iris fine white lines, which seem to lie on the surface and radiate from the pupil outward. especially in the upper part of the iris, or brain region. The signs, according to the severity of the chronic poisoning, vary from a few white lines to a thick white covering radiating from the pupil towards the upper rim of the iris (Colour plate Figs. b and e).

Cocaine.

Cocaine is an alkaloid obtained from coca leaves. The signs of this drug in the iris are similar to those of morphine. Cocaine produces local anaesthesia and anaemia by paralyzing the sensory nerves and contracting the blood vessels. When given internally in allopathic doses, cocaine acts first as a stimulant, tonic and restorative. It enables persons who chew the leaf to undergo great muscular exertion with little or no fatigue. If the use of the drug and its various preparations is continued, it has by the law of action and reaction, a paralyzing effect upon the brain and spinal cord.

I need not further dilate upon the subject of narcotics. Probably every one of my readers has come in contact with victims of these dreadful poisons, which destroy not only the body but mind and soul as well.

Anodynes and Analgesics (Pain Killers).
Sedatives and Hypnotics (Sleep Producers).

Anodynes are medicines which give relief from pain. The chief anodyne is opium, or its alkaloid, morphine. Others are canabis indica, belladonna, hyoscyamus, stramonium, conium, potassium bromide, chloral hydrate, chloroform, ether, camphor, cocaine and coal tar products. Analgesics are remedies that relieve pain, either by direct depression of the

centres of perception and sensation in the cerebrum, or by
impairing the conductivity of the sensory nerve fibres.
Antipyrine, antifebrine, phenacetin, exalgine and cocaine
are powerful analgesics. Hypnotics are medicines which produce sleep. The chief remedies of this group are bromides,
paraldehyde, sulphonal, trional, chloral hydrate, opium,
morphine, cocaine, hyoscyamus, hyoscine, ether, chloroform and alcohol.

All of these agents reduce pain and produce sleep
because they are poisonous paralyzers. They do not con-
tribute anything toward removing the causes of the pains and
insomnia; they merely benumb and paralyze the brain and
spinal centres of perception and sensation and reduce the sensitiveness and conductivity of the nerve fibres.

Natural Methods Versus "Dope".

The advocates of poisonous pain killers, nerve soothers and
sleep (?) producers have not even the excuse of lessening
human suffering. Natural methods, where it is impossible to
save life, insure at least an easy decline and painless transition. This we have proved in hundreds of cases that came to
us in the last stages of cancer and of other diseases which are
usually accompanied with great suffering. Though we have
taken care of a great many cases of cancer of the breast,
stomach, liver, intestines, etc., that came as "lost hopes" and
passed away under our care, we have administered only a few
doses of opiates to such patients within the last seventeen
years.

While ordinarily under regular treatment such sufferers
are kept constantly under the influence of opiates, and in
spite of these have to endure excruciating pain, those whom
we have treated passed through the last stages of decline
without great suffering. They all reported that their pains
were easily bearable, and, with two exceptions, none ever
asked for an opiate. The pain killers only temporarily
paralyze the sensory nerves, then pains return with increased
force. We cannot cheat nature in that or any other way. Pains
suppressed are but pains deferred. This is proved by the reactions that are sure to come after the administration of pain
killers and by the terrible tortures of the drug fiend when the

"dope" is withheld from him. Do those who administer these agents realize that they are making drug fiends of their patients before they pass from this life? We have good reason to believe that the destructive effects of these poisons continue after death. Everything in the physical has its counterpart in the spiritual. Is it not possible that the spiritual counterpart of the drug affects the spiritual counterpart of the physical body — that which St.Paul calls the "spiritual body"? Therefore, the sufferings of the drug fiend may not be ended with physical death. Every physician knows that the "dope" affects not only the physical body, but also the mental, emotional and moral characteristics; they know that the dope fiend is invariably a liar, irresponsible and unmoral. Why should a patient be exposed to such mental and physical destruction which may be of infinitely greater detriment to the permanent personality, the spiritual man, than mere physical disease, when the natural methods of treatment render the suffering easily bearable even in the most dreadful forms of chronic, destructive diseases?

In view of the fact that these poisons undoubtedly shorten the course of human life, there is another question of grave import connected with the giving of opiates. In many instances where all available vital force is needed to battle the disease, a dose of morphine or chloral may be sufficient to suppress nature's healing efforts and to bring about a fatal termination, thus robbing the patient of his last chance of recovery. Only too often the patient succumbs, not to the disease, but to the morphine syringe and other deadening hypnotics and sedatives, administered through impatience on the part of attendants and sometimes through worse motives. The last days, or even the last hours may be the most important of his life. Have we the right to deprive him of his last opportunity for retrospection and for balancing his account with the higher law?

The following incident brought this home to very forcibly. Several years ago, in one of the palatial homes of the lake shore front, I treated an old man who had amassed a great fortune, possibly not in ways exactly in harmony with the Golden Rule. He was slowly dying with cancer of the liver. His wife, forty-five years his junior, had been his faith-

ful and sympathetic nurse for several years. When the end
was near she consulted a lawyer as to the advisability of having the husband make a will in her favour. She was informed
by the legal advisor that she would be better off if no will were
made, since she was entitled to a liberal share of the fortune
as her widow's dower, and that a will might only cause trouble and complications with the many children of the testator.
From that moment on, her patience and seeming sympathy
vanished. Every word and action betrayed eagerness to see
him go. When the patient groaned with pain — or seeming
pain — she insisted that opiates be administered. Being convinced that under the natural treatment his physical suffering
was not great and that opiate would shorten his life, I
informed her that I had entered upon my life work not to take
life, but to preserve life, and that if morphine injections were
to be given some other physician must do it. The more I objec-
ted the more strongly she insisted. The patient in the meantime kept on groaning and calling for help at the top of his
voice. For hours he yelled "I am suffering terribly; something
must be done for me". Finally, at her behest, I called in a
physician who professed to be willing to administer the drug.
The patient was informed to this effect, and the doctor, ready
to apply the needle, remained within call. From that time on
until he passed away, twenty-four hours later, he never
uttered another word of complaint or a groan. He knew it
would mean the morphine syringe, and that this would shorten his life. Life was so precious to him, or possibly the dread
of the future so great, that he preferred to endure what pain
there was rather than take chances on the opiate. His
behaviour proved, as I had surmised, that his suffering was
more of a mental and spiritual than of a physical nature. Is it
not possible that the last twenty-four hours were of greater
importance to this man, as far as his spiritual welfare was
concerned, than many years of selfish grabbing and hoarding?

CHAPTER XX

DISEASES OF THE VITAL ORGANS — THEIR SIGNS IN THE IRIS

Stomach and Bowels

The area of the stomach is located directly around the pupil (A), that of the intestines surrounds the stomach (B) and the border of the intestinal field represents the sympathetic nervous system (C). See chart, Frontispiece.

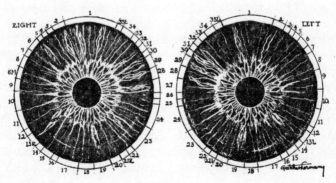

Fig. 17.

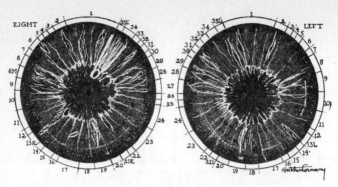

Fig. 18.

Acute conditions of these organs show white in the iris
(Fig.17), while chronic conditions, accompanied by gradual
atrophy of the membranes of these organs, create dark grey,
brown or black discolourations (Colour plate, Figs.e and f).
Acute catarrhal conditions of the stomach are usually accompanied by excessive secretion of hydrochloric acid as well as
by systemic accumulations of uric and other acids (Fig.17),
while the chronic condition, accompanied by more or less
atrophy of the membranous linings of the stomach, is responsible for deficient secretion of hydrochloric acid and pepsin
(Fig.18). In order to find out whether the contents of the
stomach are hyperacid or hypoacid, physicians of the regular
school introduce rubber tubes into the stomach and take test
samples of its contents for examination in the laboratory. The
iridologist does not have to resort to this unpleasant and
injurious practice. The showing in the iris reveals whether the
subject is suffering from hyperacidity or hypoacidity. If the
stomach area in the iris shows white, this is a sign of an acute
inflammatory and hyperacid condition, while dark discolouration indicate a sluggish, atonic or atrophic condition
of the membraneous linings and therefore a deficiency of
hydrochloric acid and pepsin. As a result of deficient secretion the foods remain undigested, enter into morbid fermentation and create noxious gases and other pathogenic materials.

If the stomach, through long continued destructive processes, is in a condition of chronic inflammation or ulceration, the inner edge around the pupil shows dark and ragged
(Fig.17). As the disease processes in the stomach proceed

from the acute and subacute to the chronic and destructive stages, we observe in the iris the appearance, first, of greyish or brownish spokes. These gradually darken until in the destructive stages they become quite heavy in appearance and black in colour (Fig. 18).

A weakened and relaxed condition of the digestive tract, resulting in enlargement and prolapsus of the organ is indicated in the iris by the distension of the areas of the stomach and bowels (Fig. 19). This is true in a more pronounced degree of the intestinal tract, which is frequently greatly distended in the areas of the caecum, ascending colon, descending colon, sigmoid flexure and rectum, these parts of the intestinal tract being frequently enlarged on account of accumulation of food materials and faeces.

RIGHT   LEFT

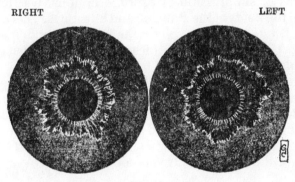

Fig. 19.

RIGHT   LEFT

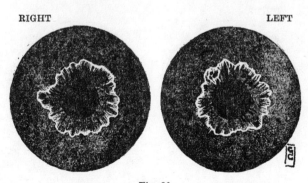

Fig. 20.

Drug Poisons in the Digestive Organs

What has been said about signs of acute and chronic conditions in the stomach is also true of the intestines. Frequently
the stomach area appears whitish, greyish or light brown,
while the intestinal area is enormously distended and shows
the black spokes of chronic conditions. In such cases stomach
digestion may be fairly active while the intestinal tract is in an
atonic condition (Fig. 19). In many cases of mercurial poisoning the intestinal area shows deep black, indicating the
paralyzing effect of the poison on the intestinal membranes.
The liver in such cases also shows chronic signs. The intestinal area frequently shows the signs of quinine, iron, sulphur, opium and its derivatives. We also find in the intestines
the signs of iodine but not of strychnine (Fig. 26). Itch spots,
the signs of suppression of psoric eruptions, we find quite
often in the fields of the stomach and intestines. These always
indicate a tendency to ulcers and benign and malignant
tumours (Fig. 20). Cancer in these organs shows usually as a
small black spot surrounded by white (Fig. 14).

(Re Fig. 20). I examined this patient six years ago and
found several large itch spots in the intestines. I informed the
husband of the lady that these itch spots indicated a strong
tendency to cancer, but she did not remain for treatment. Four
years afterwards he brought his wife to us in the last stages of
cancer of the intestines. It was too late for recovery.

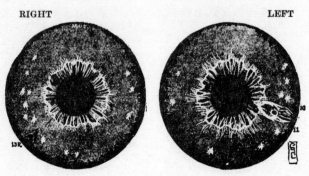

RIGHT   LEFT

Fig. 21.

(Re Fig.21). At about the same time that I made this diagnosis I examined another lady whose left breast was slightly inflamed around the nipple. Her iris revealed itch spots in the left breast. I warned her also of the possibility of cancer. She took treatment for two months; then her husband who did not believe in Natural Therapeutics, forced her to abandon the treatment and return to her home in a western city. When he brought her back three years later, the left breast was a solid mass of cancer. This case had also advanced beyond the possibility of improvement. Itch spots showed also in the left groin and liver. Mrs. S. remembered distinctly that in her childhood she had suffered with eczematous eruptions which were treated with "medicine and salves". Undoubtedly these remedies accounted for the heavy scurf rim in her eyes, and for the arsenical flakes. If these cancer patients and their relatives had understood the nature of psora and its hidden danger, both lives could have been saved.

Diseases of the Liver and Spleen

I prefer to describe these organs together because they are companion organs and we find that when one of them is seriously diseased the other also is more or less affected. These organs are the refineries of the body. The liver refines the end products of starchy and protein metabolism and discharges the waste materials thus extracted, partly in the form of bile, into the gall bladder and from there into the intestines, and partly in the form of urea which is excreted through the kidneys. It has been known to medical science that, in addition to serving as a burial ground for dead red corpuscles, the spleen has much to do with the purification of the blood, but it was not clear just how this purification took place. Many theories have been advanced which have failed to withstand the tests of scientific research and clinical experience.

The new science of Natural Therapeutics for the first time gives a rational explanation of the true function of the spleen and of the lymph nodes in the lymphatic system. This new theory has been fully explained in Chapter IX "Inflammation' in Volume I of this series and also in connection with the study of various diseases. According to this new version the spleen and the lymph nodes serve to filter the mucoid pathogenic materials out of the blood stream and to condense them into little compact bodies, the so-called leukocytes or phagocytes which have been mistaken for live, germ killing, cells. The purpose of this condensation of pathogen, as elsewhere explained, is to render the blood serum more fluid and thus to facilitate its penetration into the intercellular spaces (osmosis) and thereby the nourishment of the cells by arterial blood and their drainage by way of the lymphatic and venous systems. One of the principal reasons why Metchnikoff assumed that the leukocytes were germ killers was because they increased in numbers with the beginning of inflammation in any part of the system. He believed that they increased because more germ killers or phagocytes were needed to overcome the inflammation-creating bacteria. The new science of healing proves that inflammation takes place on account of the increase of pathogen and leukocytes, which causes obstruction in the capillary circulation. A number of serious diseases did not confirm the Metchnikoff theory. In miliary tuberculosis, malaria, typhoid fever, influenza and pernicious anaemia the leukocytes are greatly reduced in number while the spleen and nymph nodes, the capillary circulation and the intercellular spaces are blocked with leukocytes and colloid (pathogenic) materials (Fig.12, note the lymphatic rosary). The following explains this phenomenon; In these diseases the amount of pathogen in the circulation is so great that the trabeculae of the spleen and lymph nodes become so engorged with mucoid materials that they cannot any longer continue the pathogen condensing and filtering process. The failure of the spleen and lymph nodes to continue their normal functions explains the decrease in leukocytes in the circulation and the corresponding increase of colloid materials. The enlarged spleen and swollen lymph glands in quick consumption, malaria, typhoid fever, influenza and pernicious anaemia are in the same condition as a sieve that has become so clogged that it cannot any longer sift the solids from the fluids. This crowding of the lymph nodes in the neck with colloid matter can be frequently observed after the extirpation of the tonsils and adenoids, which means suppression of colloid elimination. When the lymph nodes are thus engorged with pathogenic

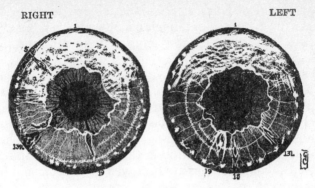

Fig. 22.

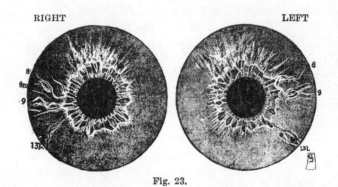

Fig. 23.

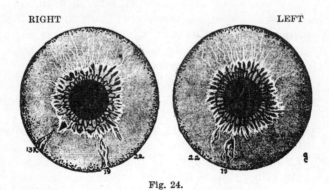

Fig. 24.

materials the surgeon knows no better than to cut them out. The practioner of Natural Therapeutics promotes the elimination of the excess of pathogenic materials from the circulation and thus relieves the engorged spleen and lymph nodules.

The foregoing explains why in serious anaemias and in other diseases before mentioned we always find in the iris the signs of acute and subacute activity in the region of the spleen and usually also in the liver, because most of the diseases of the liver also originate in pathogenic engorgement. When the colloid or mucoid obstruction in these organs continues, the acute and subacute stages are followed by chronic and finally chronic destructive stages, which is readily explained by the fact that constant pathogenic obstruction interferes with nourishment and drainage of cells and thereby brings about deterioration, degeneration and gradual destruction of the cells and tissues in the affected parts. See Series III and IV, also Fig.22-13 right and left.

Practically all diseases affecting a vital organ, whether it be the liver, spleen, kidneys, lungs, stomach or intestines, run the same course. Pathogenic obstruction first causes reaction by acute inflammatory processes. If these succeed in clearing the tissues of morbid materials, then follows recovery and normal function. If, however, the pathogenic encumbrances increase and become permanent, then the system is no longer able to remove the obstructions by acute inflammatory effort and the result is chronic degeneration and destruction (Fig.14) Series III and IV. This again confirms the teaching of Natural Therapeutics, according to which acute disease is constructive and curative in tendency while the chronic stages are characterized by atrophy and destruction of tissues. The colour of the lesions in the iris, whether they be white or greyish, brown or black, indicates what stage of pathogenic development the disease has reached.

That the ancients understood the connection between diseases of the liver and spleen and emotional conditions is proved by the fact that the word "melancholia" means "black gall". Obstruction of the gall duct is frequently caused by the accumulation of colloid materials in the form of black, tarry accretions in the gall bladder. This interferes with the flow of the bile through the gall duct into the intestine, which in turn causes the surging back of the bile into the blood stream. The absence of bile in the intestines results in constipation. Bile in the blood stream irritates brain and nerve matter, causing mental depression, melancholia or hysteria (Fig.17). I have been told on good authority that in over half the operations for gall stones no stones are found, but in place of them the black tarry substances before described — the "black gall" of the ancients. Such catarrhal obstruction of the gall duct may cause distention, painful symptoms and a bilious condition of the system, similar to that caused by obstruction by stones. Engorgement of the spleen and of the lymph nodes results in excess of pathogenic materials in the circulation. These benumb brain and nerve matter, causing physical and mental lassitude, melancholia, insanity or, in acute diseases, mental depression coma and death (Fig.18).

Cases of Chronic Quinine Poisoning
I examined Mr.L. shortly before he died of pernicious anaemia. His eyes revealed an extraordinary combination of serious lesions and signs of drug poisons, as shown in Fig.22. Lesions in the respective organs reveal a serious chronic destructive condition of the liver and gall bladder, accompanied by a collaemic, engorged condition of the spleen. The brain region, as well as the areas of liver and spleen, show distinctly the colour of quinine. In his youth he had suffered for several years with malaria, which was treated with quinine in the orthodox way. Since that time he had been affected by melancholia, indigestion, chronic constipation, neurasthenia and many other troubles, making his life a continual torture until death relieved him at the age of forty-two. His eyes also showed subacute lesions in the kidneys, several segments of nerve rings, a chronic lesion in the right ear and a closed lesion in the left knee. The pancreas area showed a large psora spot. The brain region also revealed the presence of bromides and coal tar products which had been administered to suppress the headaches and insomnia caused by quinine poisoning.

Fig.23 shows a severe lesion in the spleen and a chronic

catarrhal condition of the lungs. The patient in this case had contracted "swamp fever" in South America. After he returned to the United States this was suppressed with quinine and arsenic. The pathogenic condition of the blood caused by the diseased spleen and liver was followed by incipient tuberculosis of the lungs. Allopathic physicians admit that tuberculosis is much more dangerous when accompanied by spleen disease. Our theory of leukocytosis explains why this is so. When the circulation is saturated with excessive amounts of pathogen this will engorge and obstruct the tissues of the lungs and thus prepare the soil for tubercular processes. This patient made a perfect recovery under natural living and treatment. In practically all cases where patients told me that since they had the grippe they were troubled more or less with headaches, nervous irritability, insomnia, indigestion, bone aches, neuritis, physical and mental weakness, etc., I found in the iris the signs of quinine, indicating that the chronic after effects of influenza are not due to the disease itself but to its suppression by quinine and other poisons. This is also proved by the fact that in cases where influenza is treated by natural methods such chronic after effects never develop. Quinine shows plainly in the brain region.

Diseases of the Kidneys

The kidneys are especially prone to disease conditions because they are the filters of the system, whose function is to eliminate from the blood stream all sorts of waste and morbid materials. As long as the system is in fairly good condition and the kidneys have nothing to cope with but the normal forms of waste matter such as urea and salts, they will remain in a healthy condition, but whenever they are forced to eliminate large amounts of pathogenic materials, earthy matter, uric acid and ptomaines, bile salts, etc., the tender tissues of these organs become irritated and inflamed. This leads to morbid changes which in time render them incapable of performing their functions. When acute and subacute irritation by poisonous excretions continues for too long a time, the tissues of the kidneys undergo degenerative changes. Microscopic examination of the urine then reveals kidney cells,

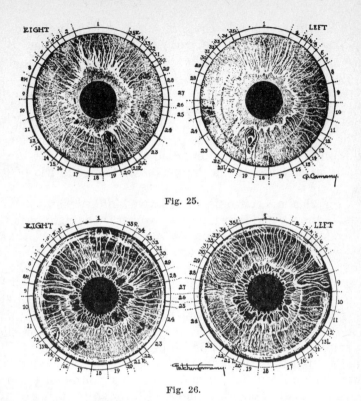

Fig. 25.

Fig. 26.

tubules, casts, leukocytes, red blood corpuscles, pus cells and other debris of inflammatory breakdown.

Fig. 24 shows both kidneys in a subacute condition. That this was not primary disease is shown by the serious lesion in the pancreas and liver which were associated with diabetes in the advanced stages. There also showed in both eyes the signs of acute inflammation in the bladder. The stomach and bowel region revealed the dark signs of chronic catarrh, indicating an atrophic condition of the membranes of the stomach and intestines, which resulted in malnutrition and systemic poisoning. The history of the patient revealed that he had been suffering from early youth with malnutrition and constipation, which I traced to the use of paregoric and cathartics. The mother of the patient told me that she had been in the habit of giving the children those wonderful "soothing syrups" and "innocent laxatives" so as not be disturbed at night or when engaged in her household duties. In the mean-time the laudanum in the paragoric and the calomel was benumbing and paralyzing the liver and intestinal membranes of her children. At the age of twenty the patient developed diabetes. This was treated with the ordinary allopathic remedies, but instead of curing the disease the poison treatment resulted in chronic inflammation and finally breakdown of the kidneys, accompanied by the discharge of albumen in addition to sugar. The patient died at the age of thirty-three, shortly after I had made the diagnosis from the iris of the eye.

Fig.25 shows chronic, destructive kidney lesions in both eyes. In the right kidney region as well as in the right back we notice large itch spots. There is a closed lesion in the left kidney and an iodine sign in the pancreas. The brain region shows the signs of acute inflammation. The patient when I examined her, was in the last stages of Bright's disease. The cause of the trouble was revealed by the itch spots. She remembered distinctly that she had had the itch several times in her youth and that it was supressed by the usual remedies — sulphur and molasses and blue ointment (mercury). She had suffered from weakness of the kidneys and bladder ever since. The poison sign in the pancreas account for the presence of sugar. The white lines all through the iris and the heavy rings indicate irritation of the nervous system through uric acid and other pathogenic materials. In this case the concentration of the psoric taint in the kidneys as the result of suppression of scabies ("seven year itch") was undoubtedly responsible for the gradual breakdown of these organs.

Stones in the Kidneys

(Fig.26). These eyes indicate plainly a uric acid diathesis. The irritation caused by this systemic poison throughout the entire system is indicated by the white lines all over the iris, giving it a grey appearance. Irritation of the nervous system by uric acid and other systemic poisons is also indicated by the many prominent nerve rings. Uric acid in this case resulted in the forming of a stone in the left kidney. This was removed by a surgical operation four years before the patient came to us for treatment. Two years after the operation another stone had formed in the right kidney. Mr. S. told me that the new stone in the right kidney was giving him much more trouble than the previous one in the left kidney; that for two years he had travelled from one hospital or sanitarium to another, his ailments growing worse all the time.

When one of a pair of organs is affected by constitutional disease and is removed by the surgeon's knife, the disease soon manifests in the companion organ. This is of such common occurrence that anyone who runs may read, but the surgeons cannot or do not want to see that constitutional disease is never cured by the mutilation or extirpation of an affected organ. Common sense reasoning would tell us that the only way to meet the problem is to cure the constitutional disease back of the trouble — in the case under discussion, the uric acid diathesis. This can easily be acomplished by natural methods of living and treatment. Before this patient came to us he developed at intervals of two weeks a violent inflammation of the affected kidney. This was accompanied by high fever and excruciating pains. The attacks, which were undoubtedly precipitated by irritation from the stone in the kidney, would last about a week and then subside, to be followed after another interval of two weeks by another attack. After he came under our care and treatment he had only one of these violent collicky attacks. After that he experienced only a few slight aggravations and improved rapidly. He left our institution five months after his arrival and, according to last reports, had not experienced another attack of kidney inflammation, but I learned from his friends that since that time he has been troubled a great deal with acute inflammatory rheumatism, which is accounted for by the fact that he was not at all strict in his adherence to the natural regimen of living. X-ray pictures which were taken just before his arrival and at the time of his departure showed that the stone had actually diminished one eighth of an inch in diameter in various directions. The acute inflammatory attacks subsided so quickly because raw food diet and fasting reduced the hyperacidity of his system very rapidly, thus lessening the irritation caused by the stone and the pathogenic condition of the blood. The fact that the stone considerably diminished in size in five months time proves that

these calculi form only in blood highly charged with acid
materials, and that they gradually dissolve under a normal
alkaline condition of the vital fluids and eliminative treatments. The digestive organs reveal a chronic catarrhal condition, also signs of iodine; in the outer margin of the iris,
deposits of salts of sodium and magnesium; subacute
catarrhal signs in bronchi, throat and nasal passages. The
chronic lesion in the rectum stands for haemorrhoids.

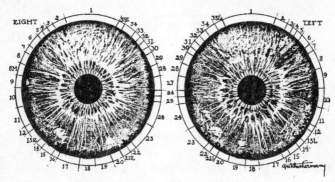

Fig. 27.

Respiratory Organs

(Fig. 27). These are the eyes of a young woman who died from
phthisis of the lungs at the age of twenty-four. I examined her
eyes three months before her death, when it had become too
late to save her life. The eyes showed the following lesions
and other abnormalities. One of the most prominent features
is a very heavy dark scurf rim which extends nearly uniformly all around the iris. This type of all-around-the-iris scurf
rim has been called by iridologists the hereditary scurf rim
because it forms early in childhood in the iris of infants who
were heavily encumbered from birth and who were subjected
to suppressive treatment for skin eruptions and other acute
infantile ailments. The application of mercurial and other
metallic ointments also results in the appearance of a broad
black scurf rim all around the iris because these metallic
poisons effectually deaden the organic structures of the cuticle. The "acquired" scurf rim is one which forms from infancy
on as the result of hot bathing, coddling, dense heavy clothing, suppressive treatment of skin eruptions. The acquired

scurf rim does not appear uniformly all around the iris but shows mainly in the form of half-moons in the outer segments of the iris (Fig. 13). The inactive, atrophic condition of the skin indicated by the heavy scurf rim predisposed the child to catarrhal conditions which manifested as whooping cough, frequent colds, profuse catarrhal elimination from the nasal passages, chronic tonsillitis and enlargement of the adenoids. At the age of four the tonsils and adenoids were extirpated. Suppression of scrofulous elimination through these channels intensified elimination through the nasal passages. The nasal membranes becoming congested, the turbinate bones soft and swollen, this obstructed the air passages and the child became a mouth breather. The nasal passages were treated with antiseptic sprays, polypi were removed and the turbinate bones reduced by the knife. This treatment resulted in destroying the nasal membrances, which suppressed the local catarrhal conditions but drove the impurities in process of elimination deeper into the system. Two years after removal of the tonsils the lymphatic glands on both sides of the neck were extirpated. About the same time the child was vaccinated before entering public school. This was followed by eczematous sores which persisted for several months and were finally "cured" by ointments and internal medication. All of this served to intensify the scurf rim.

From that time the child was never well and became pale, anaemic, weakly and listless, unable to romp and play like other children — easily tired in school, and always backward in her studies. The treatment for this anaemic condition was "good nourishing" food — plenty of meat, eggs, soups, and other heavy protein and starchy foods, which only serve to increase the pathogenic encumbrances in her system. The principal medical remedies were arsenic (Fowler's solution), strychnine and iron. Nature next tried to eliminate the pathogenic encumbrances through the bowels, which gave rise to periodic diarrhoeas. These were suppressed with laudanum and other opiates. In this fashion the child worried through the years of childhood and early youth, the parents in the meantime trying many specialists and "cures". Defective skin action and excess of protein and starchy foods intensified the pathogenic obstruction in the tissues, and resulted in carbon dioxide poisoning. This prevented the entrance of oxygen into the tissues, which meant constantly increasing oxygen starvation. This, together with pathogenic obstruction in the lung tissues, brought on constant catarrhal elimination in the form of coughing and copious expectoration. These persisted in spite of suppressive treatment by means of opiates and coal tar products, resulting gradually in the breaking down and caseous degeneration of the lung tissues, which in turn prepared a luxuriant soil for the tubercle bacilli. She was then sent to a tuberculosis camp, but the effects of the outdoor life were spoiled by stuffing with large amounts of eggs, milk and other pathogen producing foods. Death brought relief from her great suffering in her twenty-fourth year.

The eyes of this patient revealed a complete record of her progressive ailments. The areas of nose and throat showed chronic catarrhal signs and a few small closed lesions which indicated the destructive and suppressive treatment of the acute catarrhal conditions in the nose, throat, tonsils and adenoids. The neck revealed the effects of extirpation of the lymph glands. The fields of stomach and bowels to the last showed white, indicating acute catarrhal activity of those organs characterized by constant, severe diarrhoea. The areas of the lungs also showed the white signs of acute and subacute inflammation and several dark spots indicating caverns in the upper lobes of the lungs. It must be remembered that in such cases it is not only the actual destruction of tissues which brings about a fatal termination but also the pathogenic obstruction in the still active parts of the lungs. Finally, it is to be noted that the white flakes of arsenic are plainly visible in the outer portions of the iris and in the brain region the heavy grey veil of coal tar products. There are also several iodine spots. This poison was applied to the throat in a vain endeavour to "dry up" the swollen lymphatic glands. One of these spots was located in the right kidney, which showed signs of subacute inflammation.

CHAPTER XXI

CHRONIC DISEASES — THEIR SIGNS IN THE IRIS

A Case of Chronic Asthma.
(Fig.29)

Mrs. V. was brought to us five years ago, in a dying condition. She had been troubled for twenty years with asthma, digestive disorders and many other ailments. When she came to us the mucoid discharges from her throat were so copious and she was so emaciated that she presented the appearance of one labouring in the last stages of consumption. For several months it seemed that the fatal crisis might come any day. The microscope showed some tubercle bacilli in the sputum, but not enough to make it a tubercular case. After several months of natural treatment improvement came slowly but steadily. The healing crisis took the form of acute catarrhal elimination accompanied by low fever. After seven months treatment she left for home in good condition. She felt fairly well for eight months; then overwork brought on another breakdown and she returned to us for treatment. The asthmatic attacks were very distressing, and she suffered greatly from an atrophic condition of the intestines — indigestion and malnutrition, For three months she could take very little food — not more than a few spoonfuls of milk or soft boiled egg with juicy fruit or fruit juices in a day. When conditions in the alimentary tract had greatly improved a serious crisis came in the form of an acute attack of pneumonia and pleurisy. In her already weakened condition, this developed into a battle royal for life, but, as in all true healing crises, the healing forces came out victorious and from that time she improved rapidly. After this last inflammatory crisis in the respiratory organs the asthma disappeared entirely.

Mrs. V. told us that her troubles had started in childhood with stubborn constipation, indigestion and malnutrition. For this she had received allopathic treatment. She remembered that she was given considerable quantities of calomel for the liver and bowels, and strychnine and arsenic as tonics to aid digestion. When I first examined the patient her eyes distinctly showed the strychnine wheel in the stomach area and the arsenic flakes in the outer iris, especially in the lungs. These poisons, together with autointoxication and malnutrition due to her digestive troubles, probably brought on the asthmatic condition which followed in the wake of medical treatment. At the beginning of the asthmatic symptoms nature tried to relieve the respiratory organs from the morbid encumbrances by a vigorous attach of pneumonia and pleurisy. This condition also was treated in the regular way with drugs and ice packs. From that time on the asthmatic attacks increased in frequency and severity. In spite of, or probably as a result of, the continued medical treatment by the best specialists in Canada and the United States, her condition grew worse from year to year until life became a continual torture.

The sequence of healing crises, as well as her history and the records in the iris, revealed the causal chain in her case. While undergoing regeneration under the natural treatment she had to retrace the old acute diseases — the ailments that had been maltreated and suppressed in the past. The chronic conditions in the digestive organs, lungs and pleura had become acute and run their natural courses before they could be permanently eradicated. For the last few years she has been practically free from the old complaints.

When I first examined her the areas of stomach and bowels were dark brown with many black spots indicating an atrophic condition of the membranes and considerable destruction. The stomach revealed the strychnine wheel, while the intestines showed several iodine spots. She had been painted with iodine during the attack of pleurisy. The bronchi, lungs and pleura showed chronic signs of the third and fourth stages. The brain region displayed the grey, mercurial crescent; the outer margin of the iris, the whitish flakes of arsenic. The entire iris was overspread with the greyish film of coal tar products. The scurf rim was heavy and continuous all round the iris; the lymphatic rosary also was very heavy, indicating the engorged and inactive condition of the lymphatic glands. The iris picture reproduced below shows the appearance of her eyes when she first came to us five years ago. The right iris shows a lesion in the region of the knee. In her girlhood the knee was injured by a fall on the ice. The right liver area shows the sign of subacute inflammation. The chronic signs in anus and rectum (left eye), stand for external and internal haemorrhoids. At the time of writing most of the signs described and illustrated have disappeared and the iris presents a clear. blue appearance. Of the drug signs only traces of mercury and iodine are visible.

RIGHT   LEFT

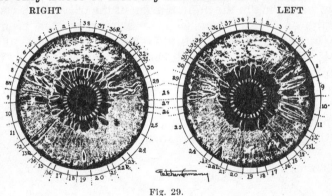

Fig. 29.

A Typical Case of Psora.
(Fig.28)

When I first met Mr. B. three years ago he had a growth on the left side of his throat the size of a large walnut. It had a soft, red spot in the centre which seemed ready to open. Several surgeons had diagnosed the case as true cancer and recommended immediate surgical removal. The eyes of this patient at the time of my first examination though apparently brown, showed on close examination a blue background. The brown, heaviest in the region of the stomach and intestines, was superimposed. When I mentioned this, he said that his mother had told him that in infancy his eyes were blue, but they had darkened and become brown when he was a few years old. The scurf rim was heavy and dark except in the brain region. The darkening of the eyes and the formation of a scurf rim must have been caused through suppressive treatment of skin eruptions, but this he did not remember and, his mother being dead, it was impossible to secure information on this point. At the age of seven he suffered with inflammatory rheumatism. This was treated by an allopathic physician. He remembered that he was confined to bed for several months and that he did not fully recover from the attack for six months. Two years later he was again prostrated with the same trouble and this time also he was not able to attend school for over six months. Since then he had been troubled periodically with rheumatism. The treatment always consisted mainly in the administration of salicylates. This accounted for the heavy white ring in the outer margin of the iris, which stands for salts of sodium, potassium and bromine, the bromine being more confined to the brain region. We always find that people who have taken salicylates repeatedly and in considerable quantities exhibit in the digestive area of the iris the brown and blackish discolourations indicating atrophy of the membranes of the gastro-intestinal tract. This patient was no exception to the rule. On being questioned he admitted that since the first attack of rheumatism he had suffered from con-

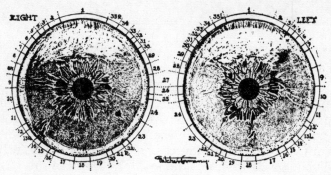

Fig. 28.

stipation and indigestion. These conditions had grown worse after the second attack and had become more chronic with advancing years. He reported that for many years he had never had a movement of the bowels without resorting to laxatives or enemas. At the age of eleven he "caught the seven year itch", as he called it. This received the regular sulphur and molasses and blue ointment treatment. It proved a stubborn case and persisted in spite of drastic treatment for about six weeks. Suppression of the scabies showed in the iris by several large itch spots, one in the right groin and one in the region of the left neck, and another in the right low back. Several smaller itch spots showed in the intestinal tract. During his childhood he was vaccinated a few times and received several antitoxin injections for immunization. This addition of disease matter to his system undoubtedly added to the vitiated condition of his vital fluids and helped to darken and discolour the iris. From childhood up he was troubled, as before stated, with stubborn constipation, indigestion and malnutrition due to the atonic condition of the intestinal membranes. Catarrhal elimination through the membraneous linings of the nasal passages, throat and bronchi endeavoured to relieve the morbid condition of his system, but he did his best to prevent this by the use of cold and catarrh cures. After his thirtieth year the rheumatism gradually became more chronic, Pathogenic obstruction in the system, together with the effects of the salicylates on the heart weakened that organ and caused it to dilate, which resulted in leakage of the mitral valve (Fig.28). At the age of foty-one a swelling appeared on the left side of the neck. It was treated first with iodine; then several doctors pronounced it to be incipient cancer and recommended immediate surgical treatment. The patient balked at this for some time. When further development of the growth left no doubt about its being of a malignant nature, he came to me for consultation and examination.

The first look in the iris revealed the large itch spot in the region of the left neck (Fig.28). I explained to him what that meant — that the psoric taint together with general autointoxication of his system was undoubedly responsible for the tumour. After a complete tracing of his ailments by the records in the iris from infancy on, he at once grasped the reasonableness of my explanations and submitted to thorough natural treatment. A description of the many crises through which he passed and their significance would fill a good sized volume. Suffice it to say that within two months after the commencement of treatment his bowels acted freely, and the skin and kidneys had become more alive and active. The first crisis came in the form of acute catarrhal elimination, which last four weeks. The thirteenth week, the second crisis brought a severe attack of acute rheumatism. This lasted for about three weeks and was followed in the fourth month by fiery, itchy eruptions all over the body. Several eczematous patches appeared on the abdomen and discharged an acrid watery fluid. The patient one day exhibited these ugly looking sores to a visiting physician who was interested in our work. The doctor could not understand why the patient seemed to be so much elated over his affliction until I explained to him that I had predicted the appearance of itchy eruptions as a form of healing crisis. I also explained the significance of the itch spots; that they stood for suppressed psora and that this constitutional taint would have to work out through acute elimination before a reduction of the malignant growth could be expected.

It is now three years since the patient ceased taking treatment. The itchy eruptions appeared and disappeared periodically, extending over a period of six months. In the meantime the tumour in the neck softened and diminished in size slowly but steadily. As the vital fluids became pure and normal the food was taken away from the parasitic growth and pure blood and lymph gradually absorbed its pathogenic materials. During the crisis periods the patient underwent three fasts of seven days, two weeks and four weeks respectively. These, together with strict raw food and at times dry food diet, aided greatly in purifying the system of its pathogenic encumbrances. Fig.28 shows the records in his eyes as they appeared when I first examined him. Note the heavy scurf rim, partly covered by the salt ring, the dark brown discolouration and black spokes in the gastro-intestinal area, standing for the atonic condition of the membranous linings of these organs caused by salicylates. The liver also shows dark, indicating a sluggish condition. The itch spots in groin, neck and intestines are plainly visible. They were dark brown in colour, indicating that the suppression had taken place many years previously. The broad white ring in the outer iris stands for deposits of salicylates. A heart lesion is plainly visible close to the sympathetic wreath in the left eye (Area 10). The upper part of the iris in the brain region shows the greyish veil of coal tar products. Iodine is visible in the left throat. The left leg had been crushed in a railway accident, which is indicated by a diagonal closed lesion.

Diabetes Mellitus.
(Figs.13-18-22-24)

The causes and rational treatment of diabetes mellitus will be described in Volume V of the series. Here I shall confine myself to a description of the signs of the disease in the iris. From the viewpoint of Natural Therapeutics we distinguish two forms of diabetes — the functional and the organic. The functional form of the disease is caused by pathogenic (mucoid) obstruction in the tissues of the body. Pathogenic obstruction prevents absorption of sugar by the cells in the muscular tissues and its combustion incidental to the performance of muscular labour. Under consumption causes excessive accumulation of sugar in the circulation, and excretion through the kidneys. If this continues for a considerable length of time, it results in the degeneration of these organs through overwork and irritation by the sugar and poisonous by-products of glycosuria such as indican, acetone, diacetic acid, ptomaines, leukomaines and other pathogenic substances. From this we see that affections of the kidneys in diabetes are, as a rule, of a secondary nature, not primary. It explains why the most serious chronic lesions appear in the pancreas, liver, stomach and intestines, while the kidneys in the initial stages of the disease exhibit signs of acure irritation. When the tendency of sugar excretion is due to pathogenic (mucoid) obstruction in the tissues of the body, then the lower half of the iris usually appears darkened while the upper half shows whitish. This indicates that the circulation is impeded in the surface, extremities and muscular tissue of the body, while the congestion exists in the larger internal arterial blood vessels in the brain, lungs and heart,

giving rise to high blood pressure. In the advanced stages of
the disease this is followed by weakness of the heart muscles
or atony of the cardiac and vasometer centres resulting in low
blood pressure. The intestinal area is usually very much distended and shows dark discolourations.

The organic form of the disease is due in most cases to
disease of the pancreas. The liver is the sugar refinery and
sugar storage house of the body. During periods of excessive
production and under consumption it stores sugar in the form
of glycogen and releases it when needed as fuel material for
the production of heat and muscular energy. The sugar
liberating activity of the liver is regulated and retarded by certain as yet obscure secretions of the pancreas; in other words,
the pancreas in this respect acts as a brake on the liver. If the
brake or regulator is out of order the liver issues more sugar
than needed. The excess accumulates in the circulation and
gives rise to glycosuria or diabetes mellitus.

Abnormal conditions of the pancreas are plainly visible
in the iris in a triangular projection from duodenum and
caecum. If the organ is normal there is nothing to be seen in
the corresponding region of the iris. If it is abnormal we
notice a triangular bulge of the intestinal wreath projecting
into areas 13 and 14 (right eye). In this triangle we find portrayed the various signs of pancreatic diseases. In many cases
I have observed the signs of acute or chronic inflammation; in
others, the signs of suppressed itch (Colour plate, fig c). In
some cases drug poisoning or suppression of psoric skin disease dated back to early infancy. Frequently such patients
strenuously deny having had itchy eruptions or eczemata or
having taken the drug shown in the iris, but careful enquiry
from relatives or the family physicians elicits the fact that the
drug had been administered for some infantile ailment, or the
skin eruptions had been suppressed during the first years of
life. It takes but very little poison to affect the tender
organism of an infant. The diagnosis from the iris is
especially valuable for detecting diseases of the pancreas.
Though frequently diseased, it is hardly ever mentioned in
allopathic and osteopathic diagnoses. The pancreas is
overlapped by the stomach and intestines, therefore if it gives
any subjective symptoms of discomfort or pain, these are

usually attributed to affections of the stomach or of the intestines, but the signs in the pancreatic triangle in the iris reveal the true nature of the trouble.

Bright's Disease

Albuminuria as well as diabetes is primarily not a kidney disease. Both ailments may be caused by degenerative changes in the kidneys, the filter organs, resulting in leakage of sugar and albumen from the blood stream. But in the majority of cases the trouble is due to abnormal constitutional conditions. As explained under diabetes these may be functional or organic. The initial phases of Bright's disease are usually caused by pathogenic obstruction of the capillary circulation and intercellular spaces. This interferes with the osmotic processes of nutrition and drainage. It prevents the consumption of proteinfood materials and causes their accumulation in the blood stream, necessitating their discharge through the kidneys. Pathogenic obstruction is gradually followed by degeneration and decomposition of the protein constituents of cells and tissue and their absorption by the blood and lymph streams. The destruction of cellular protoplasm is undoubtedly hastened by systemic acids and by drug poisons, and as it proceeds the functional stages of the disease change into the organic or destructive stages involving also the kidneys.

Pathogenic obstruction is indicated in the iris by general darkening of the colour, heavy scurf rim, white signs of acute inflammatory processes, darkening of the digestive area, nerve rings, etc. Organic destruction of tissues and organs caused by pathogenic obstruction and by the action of systemic and drug poisons is indicated by the signs of the third and fourth stages of disease. Fig.25 shows chronic deterioration in both kidneys in a case of albuminuria in the advanced stages.

Diseases of the Sexual Organs

The female sex organs are much more complicated and therefore more prone to disease than the male organs. Most of the ordinary diseases of the female sex organs have been described in Chapter XVII, entitled "Woman's Suffering", in Volume I of this series. In this chapter I shall confine myself to describing those diseases of the sex organs which are directly or indirectly due to venereal or gonnorrhoeal infection . The allopathic school teaches that these diseases are in themselves of a chronic destructive nature, and that their progress

must be stopped as soon as possible by local and constitutional treatment, by means of drugs, cauterizations,
surgical operations, etc. These teachings and practices are
erroneous and destructive. We have proved in many hundreds of cases that venereal diseases are, in themselves, of the
acute inflammatory type, that when naturally treated they
run a normal course through the five stages of inflammation
as described in Vol.I, and then leave the system in a cleaner
and more normal condition than it was before the infection.

Not a single one of these cases treated by us (before suppression had taken place) during the last seventeen years has
exhibited secondary or tertiary symptoms. As I have explained many times, it is the suppression of these diseases during the acute and subacute stages by the allopathic treatment
that causes the chronic stages and loads the system with destructive drug poisons which are responsible for the so-called
tertiary syphilis and the worst kinds of other chronic destructive diseases. Allopathy looks upon syphilis as more serious
in its after effects than gonorrhoea. Practical experience
teaches us that the reverse is true. The average gonorrhoeal
case exhibits much more painful symptoms and is more
dangerous to the neighbouring organs, as well as more destructive in its chronic after effects than syphilis. The only
reason why syphilis is followed after a lapse of years by
locomotor ataxia, paralysis agitans, paresis, and a multitude
of other so-called tertiary diseases is that slow acting but
powerful, insidious poisons are used for its suppression. The
gonorrhoeal acute catarrh of the membraneous linings of the
urethra and the syphilitic ulcer are slightly differing manifestations of the same venereal disease. This was acknowledged

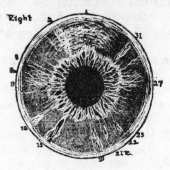

Fig. 30.

by Dr. Frankel, an allopathic specialist and writer on sexual diseases. He wrote: "The nature of the contagious poison is of minor importance. Everything depends on the more or less favourable soil the poison finds for development in the body." It sometimes happens that a gonorrhoeal infection causes syphilitic symptoms and vice versa. Nature Cure physicians claim that persons with good skin action (light scurf rim) are more prone to the gonorrhoeal form of the disease, while those with low vitality, poor skin action and of psoric constitution tend to the syphilitic form. This I have been able to verify in many instances.

In Chapter XII I have quoted at length from the writings of Dr. Joseph Hermann, who has proved, not only theoretically but by thirty years of actual practice in one of the greatest hospitals for venereal diseases in the world, that neither gonorrhoea nor syphilis are constitutional diseases; that they are easily curable in the acute stages by natural methods of living and treatment; and that all chronic and congenital after effects can be wholly avoided.

Fig.30 illustrates a typical case of gonorrhoea suppressed by injections of metallic poisons and internal medication. Area 20, urethra, and area 22, prostate gland show the signs of subacute and chronic inflammation. As in many other cases of gonorrhoeal suppression the patient is now suffering from chronic prostatitis, and the urine has to be removed by catheters. His allopathic advisers insisted upon immediate operation. This would have meant greater suffering and the beginning of the end. The suppression drove the disease taints and drug poisons into the bladder and kidneys; as a result the urine shows pus and albumen. Ever since the

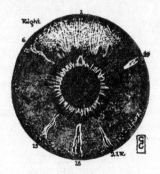

Fig. 31.

disease entered upon the subacute and chronic stages the
patient has been impotent. This is indicated by the chronic
sign in area 15, testes. During the subacute stages the right
wrist became affected with gonorrhoeal arthritis; this was
also suppressed and left the joint in an ankylosed condition
(area 12). It is a peculiarity of gonorrhoeal arthritis that it
affects only one joint at a time. The gonorrhoeal taint in the
system will aggravate any tendency to rheumatism and make
it more malignant. Suppression of the acute catarrhal
elimination from the urethra resulted in chronic catarrh of the
nasal passages and bronchi. This, in turn, was treated and
suppressed for years with coal tar poisons. As a result of long
continued drug poisoning, especially by salicylates administered for rheumatism and arthritis, the area of stomach and
bowels show chronic catarrhal signs, indicating indigestion,
chronic constipation, gas formation and malnutrition. Of special interest in this is the quinine sign in the brain region
especially prominent in area 2, right cerebellum, which is the
seat of sex life, the emotional nature, etc. The patient con-
fided to me that from early youth he had suffered with
excessive excitation of the sex impulse. Undoubtedly this
was caused by quinine taken in considerable quantities for
chills and fever during his sixth and seventh years.

Fig. 31 illustrates the right eye of a woman fifty years old,
who, at the age of twenty-five, contracted a syphilitic infection from her husband. The doctor who treated her, in order to
shield the husband, did not inform her of the true nature of the
disease. Not until she studied natural methods of healing and
became a drugless healer herself did she find out the true
cause of her ailments. When she came to me for treatment she
exhibited a hole in the palate as large as a dime, which communicated with the nasal passage. This lesion did not develop
until many years after the syphilitic ulcer had been suppressed with mercury and potassium iodide. The inguinal
glands and ovaries had been affected at the time by swellings
(bubo) and inflammation. When I examined her, both areas
(15,18) in the iris showed chronic signs and a large iodine spot
in the right bladder. The patient informed me that after the
suppression of the original acute condition she had lost sexual sensation. The fields of the lower extremities reveal the
signs of subacute inflammation. This was treated for years as
sciatic rheumatism with salicylates and painkillers (narcotics
and opiates). Subsequent developments showed that the sup-

posed sciatic rheumatism marked the first stages of locomotor ataxia caused by the action of mercury and potassium
iodide on the lower spinal cord. The upper part of the iris
shows distinctly the greenish crescent of mercury. Iodine is
visible in areas 28, 23, 10. Area 29, neck, shows signs of subacute inflammation due to engorgement and inflammation of
the lymphatic glands. The brain region exhibits acute signs in
cerebrum and cerebellum. The accompanying symptoms are
frequent headaches and dizziness. The patient under natural
treatment experienced great improvement. The hole in the
palate healed over perfectly within four months time. Her
general condition improved sufficiently within six months for
her to be able to resume her work as a drugless practitioner.

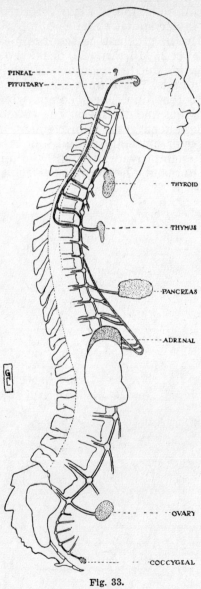

Fig. 33.

CHAPTER XXII

THE DUCTLESS GLANDS AND THEIR SECRETIONS
(Fig. 33)

The secretions of the ductless glands are called internal secretions because they are not carried to the exterior by an open duct, but are poured directly into the blood and lymph. Certain glands with ducts have also internal secretions, as for instance, the pancreas. In fact, it is claimed by some authorities that every specialized tissue in the body produces secretions which in some way influence the vital activities. From this it becomes apparent that internal secretion is one of nature's methods of coordinating the activities of the various parts of a complex organism. The more easily understood coordination, by means of the nervous system, is of later development in the evolutionary process. In the following paragraphs I shall briefly describe the locations and functions of the ductless glands, and follow with a summary of the teachings of Dr. Charles E. de Sajous concerning the coordination and functions of these interesting organs.

1. Pineal Gland. This is a small body projecting from the roof of the third ventricle at the base of the brain, beneath the corpus callosum. It is glandular in structure, reaching maximum development about the seventh year. After this period and particularly after puberty it degenerates into fibrous tissue. It contains a few atrophied nerve cells without axons. Occultists claim that all through life this gland is in active communication with the pituitary glands; that, in fact, the life impulses pass from the pineal gland into the pituitary bodies and from these and the nervous system all through the organism. Disease of this gland results in a too rapid development of the reproductive organs and upon the growth of the skeleton.

The pineal gland is better developed in the hatteria (lizards) and lamprey (fishes) than in man. In these lower animals it is often found in duplicate organs. One of these organs then corresponds to the gland proper, while the other develops into an eye-like structure connected by nerve fibres to the habendula ganglia. This third eye is situated centrally on the upper surface of the head but is covered with skin. An ancient myth tells about human beings who possessed a third eye at the back of the head.

2. Pituitary Gland This glandular structure is situated in the sella turcica of the sphenoid bone, at the base of the brain. It consists of three parts which are structurally and functionally different:

(1) Anterior Lobe;

(2) Pars intermedia. This corresponds to the "test organ" of Sajous;

(3) Posterior Lobe, developed from the floor of the third ventricle. In adults it consists mainly of neuroglia.

Hypertrophy of the anterior lobe results in acromegaly or enlargement of the bones of the face and limbs. Partial removal causes increase of adipose tissue and atrophy of the sexual organs (sex infantilism).

3. Thyroid Gland. This ductless gland consists of two oval lobes lying one on each side of the windpipe, just below the Adam's apple, and connected by an isthmus or middle lobe. Absence or atrophy of the gland in children causes cretinism (idiocy). Removal or atrophy of the gland in adults causes myxoedema. The organ secretes iodothyrin which contains 9.3 percent iodine by dry weight. Since perverted nitrogenous metbolism invariably follows complete removal of the thyroid gland, it is evident that this gland must supply the system with some principle which enables it to assimilate nitrogen for repair and to oxidize nitrogenous waste products prior to their elimination.

4. Parthyroids.   These structures consist of four oval bodies, two on each side of the thyroid gland, from which they differ in structure and function. Complete removal results in acute toxic symptoms which develop rapidly. The most prominent is muscular tetany.

5. Adrenals.   The adrenal glands are situated on top of the kidneys. Adrenalin ($C_9H_{13}NO_3$) is the basic substance in the secretions of these organs. The secretions of these glands are increased in a marked degree by fear, rage or other emotional excitement. The injection of adrenalin produces general vasoconstriction of the blood vessels. Degeneration or atrophy of the adrenals causes Addison's disease, dark pigmentation of the skin, muscular weakness, low blood pressure, mental apathy and general wasting.

6. Reproductive Glands.   These are the testes of the male and the ovaries of the female. In these organs are located, in addition to the sex cells, the cells of Leydig outside of the seminal bodies. Complete castration in young males arrests development. Transplantation of testes to some other part of the body in animals is followed by normal development in sexual desire and potency. Substitution of ovaries for testes in young males arrests development of male genitals and the animal finally acquires all the instincts and characteristics of the female. The internal secretions of the sex glands are important not only as regards the so-called secondary sexual characteristics, but also have a very marked stimulating effect upon all processes of oxidation in the system.

7. Thymus Glands.   This organ is situated behind the upper part of the sternum at the base of the neck. It was formerly supposed to reach maximum development at birth and subsequently to atrophy. Recent observers claim, however, that it continues to increase in size after birth until the coming of puberty, and it may persist through life. Castration results in the persistent growth of the thymus gland. Removal of the thymus hastens the development of testes or ovaries. Thymus fed to dogs stimulates the growth of the body but results in mental deterioration. Thymus fed to young tadpoles retards bodily growth but hastens metamorphosis, thereby producing dwarf frogs. It is claimed that thymus extract prevents excessive accumulation of acids, particularly of the acid of phosphorus, which it neutralizes into nuclean compounds. Thymus, therefore, seems to stimulate physical growth and to retard mental growth.

8. Coccygeal Gland. This small gland lies in front of the tip of the coccyx. Its removal is followed by serious nervous disturbance.

9. Carotid Gland. This gland is located at the bifurcation of the common carotid arteries. Its exact functions are also unknown as yet, but both the coccygeal and the carotid glands seem to act as neutralizers of systemic poisons.

The Relationship of the Ductless Glands.

Until a few years ago little or nothing was known about the functions of the ductless glands in animal and human bodies. Probably physiologists and physicians would still be describing these structures as "atrophied organs", the relics of a previous and now utterly changed anatomy of man during some period of his evolutionary development, had not some surgeons, regarding these organs as atrophied and useless relics of the past, extirpated them and found that people thus deprived of these "useless relics" invariably developed serious chronic diseases of body or mind, or even died. Now, certain branches of advanced medical science jump to the other extreme and attribute practically all diseases to the abnormal functioning of these small and seemingly insignificant organs.

Sajous has probably done the most advanced work along these lines of physiological and medical research. The substance of his "theory and practice" as presented in the "Internal Secretions and Principles of Medicine", may be summarized as follows: "The pituitary body or gland (Fig.33), acting through the sympathetic and central nervous systems and through the thyroid and adrenal glands, controls all the vital processes of the body." Thus modern materialistic science meets and corroborates ancient esoteric science, which taught, in what we are pleased to call the "dawn of humanity", that the pineal gland and pituitary bodies were the organs of the spirit and the soul through which the life forces act upon the body. Concerning the relationship and various functions of these organs, Sajous says: "the pituitary body is the general and governing centre of the spinal system, which includes the grey substance at the base of the brain, the pons and spinal cord, and the nerves derived from any of these structures, cranial and spinal. The pituitary body is the governing centre of all vegetative functions, i.e., of the somatic brain. The pituitary gland is divided into an anterior and posterior body. The anterior is a lymphoid organ which, through the posterior body and a nerve path in the spinal cord, governs the functional activity of the adrenals. Since the secretions of the adrenal glands control all the oxidation processes of the body, this control is exercised originally from and through the anterior pituitary body. In like manner the anterior pituitary body governs, by means of the posterior body and certain nerve tracts, the activity of the thyroid gland. The pituitary body, the adrenals and the thyroid gland are thus functionally united, forming the adrenal system. The posterior pituitary body is the seat of the highly specialised centres which govern all the vegetative or somatic functions of the body, or of each organ individually. The posterior pituitary body receives all the sensory impressions belonging to the field of common sensibility; pain, touch, muscular sense, etc., initiated in any organ, including the mucous membrane of skin and brain." (According to this the pituitary bodies must be the organs through which the consciousness receives impressions from without and within.) "The sympathetic nervous system is also governed by a highly sensitive centre likewise located in the posterior pituitary body. The 'sympathetic centre' in the posterior pituitary body through the sympathetic system governs the calibre of all arterioles and regulates the volume of blood admitted into the capillaries of any organ, including those of the brain and nervous system. The calibre of the larger blood vessels is governed through the vasomotor centre."

The Test Organ.
"Between the two lobes of the pituitary body is located an organ which has for its purpose the protection of the individual against morbid and poisonous materials which may be present in the circulation. This test organ reacts to the

influence of any poison capable of exciting it. It reacts to such morbid and poisonous stimuli by increasing the functional activity of the thyroid and the adrenal glands. By increasing the functions of the adrenals it enhances the antitoxic powers of the blood and of the phagocytes. The secretions of the thyroids and parathyroids jointly form the obsonin and glutinin of the blood" (Substances which serve to devitalize disease producing bacteria).

From the foregoing it follows that the adrenal system, composed of the pituitary body, the adrenals and the thyroid apparatus, constitute the detoxifying and immunizing mechanism of the body. Inasmuch as the adrenal system has for its purpose the protection of the body against disease, it is by enhancing the functional activity of the adrenal system that we can overcome disease. The "vis mediatrix naturae" is due to the presence of auto-antitoxin, i.e., obsonin and other antibodies, in the circulation. As to the normal functions of the adrenals (thyroid and adrenals) during health, Sajous says: "The adrenals supply an internal secretion which absorbs the oxygen of the air and carries it to the tissues". This secretion of the adrenals he calls "adrenoxidase". On this oxidase depends pulmonary and tissue respiration. The red blood corpuscles are storage cells for adrenoxidase. The adrenal secretion is the one ferment which imparts to all other body ferments their particular properties. All these propositions seem to be well proven. Extensive experimentation and clinical experiences seem to prove the main facts herein described. But when Sajous comes to the therapeutic part of his philosophy of disease and cure he cannot get away from the orthodox allopathic idea of poison treatment. All through his therapeutic deductions and suggestions he tries to fit in the allopathic materia medica and artificial antitoxin treatment with the wonderful activities of the pituitary centre and the ductless glands. He endeavours to show that mercury, iodine, quinine and the host of other poisonous drugs exert a curative action by stimulating the pituitary bodies and, through these, the other ductless glands. He claims that through the stimulating effect of these poisons the secretions of thyroid and adrenals are gradually increased and that thereby the auto-antitoxins in the circulation becomes more abundant and more active. From this we see that his idea of treatment is still symptomatic. Although he recognizes that the processes of inflammation and fever are constructive, his treatment is symptomatic in so far as he ignores the pathogenic substances in the system which in the first place benumb the adrenal system — the protective mechanism of the body. If he would concentrate his therapeutic efforts upon preventing the creation of these toxic pathogenic substances and upon their elimination from the system by harmless natural methods, then the protective mechanism of the body — the pituitary and other ductless glands — would revive spontaneously and become more alive and active. Instead, he has nothing to say about the prevention of pathogenic processes nor about the elimination of disease producing materials through natural methods of treatment. The sum and substance of his treatment consists either in stimulating the ductless glands into greater activity by the most virulent and destructive poisons on earth, or in administering substitutes for the glandular secretions in the form of glandular extracts from animal bodies. What the drug poisons do to the system later on is not his concern. The fact that they create the most destructive chronic diseases has not yet dawned upon his "scientific mind".

These recent discoveries of the importance of the pituitary bodies, which practically reveal them as the seat of the life force which intelligently controls the manifold vital processes, are an interesting corroboration of the teachings of esoteric science, which describes the pineal and pituitary glands as the organs through which the spiritual and psychical forces act upon the body and create the various planes of consciousness in man. The pineal gland is that which the occultists call "Devaksha". the "Divine Eye". It is the chief organ of spirituality in the human brain, the seat of genius, the mythical sesame for the purifying of the mystic, that which opens all the avenues of truth for him who knows how to use them. According to these teachings, the pineal gland is, during life, connected with the pituitary bodies and through these with the physical material organism.

Organo Therapy.

When the old school of medicine began to realize the impor-

tance of the secretions of the ductless glands and of other
organs and membranes in the vital processes of the body, they
attempted to supply these secretions in certain diseases of the
ductless glands by administering the corresponding glandular
organs, or extracts of these organs, from animal bodies. Thus
they extracted pepsin, the digestive principle of gastric juice,
from the stomachs of animals. In like manner they prepared
extracts of the pituitary glands, thymus and thyroid glands,
adrenals, pancreas, portions of the intestines and of other
organs and membranes, and administered them as substitutes
for the like tissues or secretions of the human body. Until a
few years ago pepsin was held to be a certain and sure remedy
for indigestion, but in all my experience I have yet to come
across a single patient who has been cured of digestive trouble by this preparation. It is true that these animal extracts, in
many cases, act as palliatives; but I have never found them
curative. The reason for this is obvious. We cannot strength-
en a feeble arm by carrying it in a sling. Crutches do not cure
the paralyzed limb nor do glasses always cure weak eyes. The
great law of use ordains that any faculty, capacity or power —
physical, mental or moral — which we do not constantly use
and exercise, weakens and atrophies. Animal extracts, and
all other kinds of crutches favouring and substituting certain
organs and functions of the human organism, do not
strengthen these nor reestablish lost functions, but through
taking away the natural stimuli and preventing natural use
and excercise, the organs thus favoured become more lazy,
benumbed and atrophied.

Natural Therapeutics follows the opposite plan. In the
first place, it corrects the primary causes of disease which
were responsible for the weakening and degeneration of the
secreting glands and membranes; then it makes these more
active and alive through hydrotherapy, massage, neurotherapy and magnetic treatment, through curative gymnastic
exercise, sun baths and other natural methods of treatment. I
do not remember a single case of soft goitre that we have not
cured without the use of thyroid extract. In like manner we
have cured other so-called chronic, incurable diseases supposed to be caused by a deficiency of glandular secretions,

At best the correct selection and administration of these

endochrine preparations is very difficult and even dangerous. This is admitted by the best medical authorities. Why should we resort to these uncertain agents when natural methods of treatment do work without risk? I can imagine cases of extreme urgency where the administration of such preparations may be advisable as a temporary palliative and substitute until the natural secretions can be made to flow. But it is certain that continued administration of these substances will delay or prevent the natural production of the secretions. The best proof of this is that the great majority of patients coming to us for treatment of goitre, of digestive troubles or disease of the adrenals, have taken the animal extracts for years without attaining permanent satisfactory results. Each told the same story. At first the glandular extract seemed to bring about great improvement, but this was soon followed by relapse into the former chronic condition. How can it be otherwise? The beneficial effects of the animal extracts are soon offset by the progress of the disease which caused the atrophy of the ductless glands or secreting membranes in the first place. For instance, the membraneous linings have been ruined by hyperacidity and general toxicity of the system. The pepsin cells have become impaired, thus causing indigestion. Animal pepsin, administered as a substitute, for a time brings improvement, but the disease conditions continue to grow worse and weaken, not only the stomach, but other organs as well. In this way the temporary improvement brought about by the pepsin is gradually offset and overcome by the general decline of the system.*

*Since Lindlahr's death a system of so-called Endogenous Endocrinotherapy has been developed and advocated by Dr. Jules Samuels of Amsterdam. This system is based on the spectroscopic diagnosis of the performance of the principle endocrine glands (particularly the pituitary, thyroid and gonads) and the restoration of a proper balance between them by stimulation of glands which are under-functioning and control of those which are over-functioning. The treatment which is used is founded on the use of short-wave radiations and there is evidence that it is highly successful. Moreover it would seem to be free from the objections voiced by Lindlahr to other forms of endocrine therapy including the use of hormonal preparations derived from animals. This is because it aims at restoring normal and balanced functioning of the endocrine system as a whole and not merely at making up for a deficiency of a particular hormone, which is at best a palliation rather than a cure. When a satisfactory balancing of the endocrine system has once been attained it will have a strong tendency to remain because the glands are correlated and regulate each other when they are functioning normally. It should be mentioned that a friend and colleague of mine, Mr. L.R. Ogden, now deceased, working on the basis of Samuel's method, claimed to have had success in greatly simplifying it both in diagnosis and in treatment. He carried out the diagnosis by electronic means and the treatment by sonics.

CHAPTER XXIII

DISEASES OF THE DUCTLESS GLANDS — THEIR SIGNS IN THE IRIS

Hyper-Thyroidism or Goitre.
(Fig.32)

The thyroid gland is a double lobed gland, connected by a narrow bridge, situated in front of and on both sides of the trachea at the base of the neck. It is now proved that the secretion from this gland has much to do with the oxidation and absorbtion of protein food materials. It provides the blood with a substance which enables the body to assimilate nitrogenous food elements and to oxidize and eliminate protein waste and morbid materials. Goitre is an ailment characterized by permanent enlargement of the thyroid gland. This is usually accompanied by accelerated and irregular heart action and by more or less pronounced and serious nervous symptoms. The secretions of the thyroid are tonic in their action and act as a strong stimulant when present in large quantities. The gland has an abundant blood supply and becomes enlarged very readily when unduly irritated by systemic or drug poisons. The disease is very common in Switzerland and certain other parts of Europe. It has been attributed to excessive amounts of lime in the drinking water, but this does not hold true in all cases. Heredity and excess of protein in the diet are undoubtedly prominent factors.*

Soft Goitre.
(Fig.32, Area 28, right)

In the first stages of this disease the enlargement is soft and spongy, but in time it becomes tough and hardened until it appears to the touch like hard rubber. The enlargement in the soft stages is due to some kind of irritation and over-stimulation. When the source of this irritation or over-stimulation is removed through natural living and treatment, the enlargement is readily absorbed and disappears entirely within a few months.

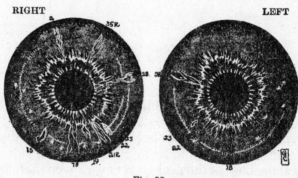

RIGHT   LEFT

Fig. 32.

*Lindlahr here mentions the undoubted fact that there are certain localities or "goitre belts" where the incidence of goitre is very high and can almost be described as endemic, but he does not seem to lay great emphasis on the importance of this or to explain its significance. There can be little doubt that the reason for the existence of goitre belts is that in these areas there is a deficiency of iodine in the soil and that this leads to a failure in the normal production of thyroxin. Though Lindlahr may be right that goitre is generally due much more to over-stimulaton of the thyroid by nitrogenous wastes and poisons in the circulation or by spinal lesions there must be many cases in which iodine deficiency is playing a part to a greater or lesser degree. This deficiency when it does exist should be corrected by the right kind of treatment of the soil, as, for instance, the use of seaweed as an organic fertilizer. Iodine is one of the elements of which the body has need but it is not a thing which should be supplied in inorganic form whether as a dietary supplement or as a medicament, in spite of the fact that it is widely used by doctors for the prevention or threatment of thyroid troubles.

Lindlahr in his discussion of iodine earlier in this volume shows very convincingly how harmful the use of inorganic iodine can be and he was dead against the use of iodized salt. He maintains that the long term effects of such practices are bound to be bad even if in the short term there may be some symptomatic improvements. It is along the lines of all round natural treatment that thyroid troubles should be approached.

Hard Goitre.

Long continued irritation, over-stimualation, acute and chronic inflammation are always followed in time by atrophy of the affected organs and by the formation of connective or scar tissue. This occurs in the thyroid gland after prolonged irritation and over-stimulation. The soft enlargement then gradually turns into hard connective tissue similar to a fibrous tumour. After this has been in existence for some time even strict adherence to natural methods of living and of treatment may not succeed in dissolving and absorbing these hard formations. In such cases, however, natural treatment will result in purifying the body, adjusting mechanical lesions and in improving the vital processes, thus restoring the system as a whole to as good a condition as is possible in the circumstances.

Ever since I began to teach the principles of natural healing I have claimed that enlargement of the thyroid gland was caused in most cases through irritation of the organ by systemic or drug poisons. When the circulation becomes overcharged with nitrogenous waste and systemic poisons the gland enlarges and its secretions become more profuse. Excessive secretion over-stimulates the nervous system and heart action and causes increased oxidation (destruction) of protein waste and also of protein tissues and food substances. This, in turn, produces loss of flesh and weight. The succeeding gradual atrophy of the glandular tissues tends to inhibit the hyperactivity of the organ and is followed in time by the opposite condition of deficient secretion. While the natural dietetic treatment is very much the same in both extremes of soft and hard goitre, the manipulative treatment must be entirely different. In the first soft and hyperactive stages the nerve and blood supply of the gland should be inhibited. In the atrophic stages the treatment must be stimulative in its effects.

Over-stimulation of the thyroid gland frequently occurs through toxins produced by some septic disease, but in such cases the increased secretions from the gland may be needed to neutralize the toxic materials generated by the inflammatory processes; in other words the hyperactivity of the thyroid is protective and will diminish as the disease subsides. Irritation and over-stimulation of the gland may also be caused through spinal lesions. Luxated bones, strained muscles or ligaments may irritate the nerves which supply the thyroid and thus cause hyperactivity of the organ. We have cured many soft goitres by removing such mechanical irritation by neurotherapy treatment.

Exopthalmic Goitre or Grave's Disese.
(Fig.32, Area 28, right)

This is an aggravated form of goitre, accompanied by increased rate of heartbeat, muscular tremors, etc. It derives its name from a characteristic symptom — protrusion of the eyeballs. This as well as the peculiar stare which it produces is caused by excessive nerve and blood pressure from within. The disease is more common in women between the ages of fifteen and thirty, and in men between thirty and forty-five. Nervous shock, grief, fright and over-taxation of the nerves are exciting and contributing causes. The pulse is sometimes as high as 200 per minute. The patient is very often anaemic, the heart becomes hypertrophied as a result of its rapid and violent action, which is very often followed by dilatation, including leakage through improper closing of the valves. Palpitation of the heart is a frequent symptom, as also is the staring look caused by protrusion of the eyeballs, which may be accompanied by other ocular disturbances, such as paralysis of the lids, or paralysis of one or more of the nerves controlling the action of the eyeballs. The thyroid gland itself is moderately enlarged at first and rather soft and elastic, but it becomes harder and firmer as the result of the proliferation of connective tissue. Muscular tremor is common and may affect the whole body or only the limbs. Other symptoms may be present, such as digestive disturbances, kidney involvement inducing excessive formation of urine or showing the presence of sugar or albumin in the urine, occasional fever, skin eruptions, mental depression, melancholia or mania. In all cases of goitre we find that the urine contains excessive amounts of indican, skatol, indol and phenol, and other forms of ptomaines and leukomaines created through putrefactive changes in the intestines and other parts of the body. This indicates the source of the trouble, namely, excessive produc-

tion of poisonous acids and alkaloids of putrefaction resulting from unbalanced diet and defective elimination through
clogging and atrophy of the skin, bowels and kidneys.
Pathogenic materials and drug poisons over-stimulate the
thyroid and other ductless glands. Continued hyperactivity
and increase of secretions from the thyroid and adrenals not
only results in excessive oxidation of protein food materials,
but also in destruction of fleshy tissues of the body. This, in
turn, increases nitrogenous waste and alkaloids of putrefaction, and these will cause complete prostration and death
unless the destructive processes are arrested. The toxic condition of the system and increase of thyroid secretion over-
stimulates the nervous system and heart action, causing high
frequency of the pulse.

Treatment.

The patient should be treated upon the appearance of the first
symptoms. The increased function of the thyroid gland in this
disease may be caused by insufficiency of the internal secretions on the part of the suprarenals, ovaries, testes or
pituitary gland. Consequently it requires general treatment
for the purpose of toning up the entire body. The cardiac
symptoms, when they are severe, can be relieved by careful
manipulative treatment of the spine. Fresh air, moderate
exercise and rest, are required to make a good recovery. No
attempt should be made to suppress the activity of the thyroid
gland itself by painting with iodine or by the use of ice bags,
X-ray or other powerful suppressive agents. The diet at first
should be directed toward increasing elimination and consequently should consist largely of fruits and vegetables, and
later may be extended to include a moderate amount of protein (grains, nuts, milk and, occasionally, eggs). Massage and
Swedish movements must make the organs of elimination
more alive and active. The spinal lesions must be corrected
through neurotherapy treatment; open air exercise, sun and
air baths, constructive attitude of mind and soul, all must
combine to produce normal conditions, physically and mentally. As this is being accomplished, the thyroid gland as well
as all other organs in the body will gradually become normal
in structure and function.

Allopathic Treatment.

Allopathy, in accordance with its general trend of theory and practice, attributes these diseases of the thyroid gland to infection from other foci of inflamation, such as diseased tonsils, adenoids, abscesses in the teeth, ovaries or other parts of the body. The "Handbook of Therapy", edited by the American Medical Association, says under "Hyperthyroidism": "The aetiology of hyper-thyroidism is not yet determined . . . . There are numerous reports in the literature of cases of hyper-thyroidism (goitre) following acute or chronic infections such as tonsilitis, sinusitis, arthritis and salpingitis. These facts make it seem likely that the disease is due to metastatic infection of the thyroid gland. The treatment of hyper-thyroidism is based on two main factors. First, alleviation of symptoms; and second, removal of the foci of infection which may be responsible". This means, of course, that the symptoms — nature's healing efforts — must be suppressed, and the foci of infection in other parts of the body must be removed through suppressive antiseptic, germicidal or surgical treatment.

Natural living and treatment will remove the foci of infection in the teeth, tonsils, ovaries, appendix, or wherever they exist, in exactly the same rational and efficient manner in which it cures all other ailments of the body. Bromides and coal tar poisons for the excited brain and nerves, cathartics for the sluggish bowels, and paralyzing sedatives for the rapid heart may be good "symptomatic" treatment, but they do not touch the underlying causes of the trouble.

More destructive than the symptomatic drug and serum treatments are the more radical iodine, surgical and Roentgen Ray treatments. These are positively destructive in their effects upon the system. We have learned from our study of iodine in Chapter XIV that this poison atrophies glandular structures all through the body. This explains the action of the poison in the treatment of goitre. Painted on the throat, it is absorbed and atrophies the glandular structures of the thyroid. Iridiagnosis proves, however, that the poisons applied to the throat usually locates in other parts or organs — a lucky thing for the thyroid. Fig.31 illustrates this fact. It shows the iodine in the lower back and chest as well as in the thyroid. Understanding the importance of this little organ in the vital functions, what a dangerous procedure this is. As already stated, the iodine absorbed into the circulation may affect other organs or glandular structures in the system such as mammary glands, the adrenals, ovaries, testes, etc., and destroy their fuctions. Later on, the red spots of iodine clearly reveal in the iris of the eye where the poison has accumulated in the body. In my own case, as I have related elsewhere in this volume, the iodine rubbed into my throat in order to reduce enlarged lymphatic glands happened to concentrate in liver and kidneys, thus laying the foundation for chronic disease of these organs. Incidentally, it was the iodine poisoning which helped to bring me into this work.

Surgery for Goitre.

The surgical treatment consists in snipping off parts of the enlarged organ, I suppose with the idea of reducing its hyperactivity. I can find only one fitting adjective for describing such unnatural treatment, and that is the word "criminal". Such wilful destruction can never be compensated. If total extirpation of the organ is surely followed by death within a few days, why destroy part of it? We know positively that natural living and treatment will restore the little organ to a normal condition (if destruction has not too far advanced), but it cannot restore that which has been destroyed by the surgeon's knife. I have had occasion to observe a number of cases that have been operated on and all of them developed, sooner or later, serious chronic constitutional diseases. Some drifted into tuberculosis, others developed malignant tumours or died from malassimilation and malnutrition, still others developed serious nervous conditions, several became insane. Several years ago a patient of mine tried to induce a friend to have natural treatment for exopthalmic goitre instead of submitting to an operation. But the patient and her friends had more confidence in their "great specialist" than in Nature Cure. The ends of the thyroid were snipped off and within twenty-four hours afterwards the lady was completely paralyzed on one side. Death ended her sufferings about two years after the operation.

Thyroid Deficiency.
(Fig.32, Area 28, left)

The opposite of the conditions described under hyper-thyroidism we find in cases where for some reason or another the thyroid fails to produce a sufficiency of secretions. Where this condition is caused by defective development of the gland from birth, it results in cretinism. This word is derived from the French word "cretin", meaning "dwarf". Cretinism therefore signifies backward development both physically and mentally. The child is dwarfed and very ugly. The tongue is too large for the mouth, and the voice is harsh and squeaky. The hair is coarse, the abdomen prominent, hernia is common. The sexual organs remain undeveloped, so do also the mental functions, and the vocabulary is very limited. A few cases reach adult life, but the majority die in childhood. The regular medical treatment consists in the administration of thyroid extract daily throughout life.

Better and more permanent results are obtained by thorough, all round Natural Therapeutic treatment. The diet must be carefully regulated. The little patient must receive a generous supply of the positive mineral elements. Careful massage and neurotherapy treatment, consisting largely in stimulation of the nerve centres which supply the thyroid gland, has a wonderfully vivifying effect in such cases. Magnetic treatment also is very beneficial in this as well as in all other forms of thyroid disease. Cold water treatment, sun and air baths, and the indicated homoeopathic remedies all help to make the dormant organ more alive and active. I always find that the plastic, sensitive organisms of children and infants respond much more readily to the natural influences than the coarser and more heavily encumbered bodies of adults.

Thyroid deficiency in adults may result from many different causes. Pathogenic matter may clog or benumb and paralyze the glandular structures. Poisonous drugs may produce similar results more quickly. The nerve supply of the gland may be greatly interfered with by luxated spinal vertebrae or through pressure on the nerves by contracted or strained muscles, ligaments or connective tissue growth.

While hyperactivity of the gland often results in great

emaciation, deficiency of thyroid secretion tends to cause the opposite condition, namely, obesity or excessive flesh and fat formation. This in itself proves that the secretion of the thyroid promotes the processes of oxidation. One of the principal causes of excessive fat formation lies in the defective oxidation of protein, starchy and fatty materials. In such cases small doses of thyroid extract, carefully regulated, help to reduce excessive fat formation. This treatment is at best only palliative, the underlying causes of the ailment must be overcome by natural living and treatment. Natural diet and treatment must bring about greater activity of the organ and improve the processes of digestion and elimination.

Symptoms Peculiar to Diseases of the Thyroid Gland. Many people suffer more or less all their lives from severe headaches which defy all sorts of treatment. A great deal of this life-long torture is due to either temporary or constant inactivity of the thyroid gland. Deficiency of thyroid elements in the circulation with the oxidation of food materials as well as of systemic poisons, causing, on one hand, nerve starvation, and on the other hand, brain and nerve poisoning. (See nerve rings, Fig.32, left and right.) We have cured many such cases in individuals who had suffered all their lives either at intervals or continuously with headaches resulting from such causes. The accumulation in the system of nitrogenous waste due to insufficient activity of the thyroid also becomes frequently one of the contributing factors in asthma and in other chronic diseases of the respiratory organs. The pathogenic materials in the circulation are not oxidized and eliminated from the system on account of the deficiency of thyroid and adrenal secretions in the blood. Therefore they accumulate in the circulation and clog and benumb the tiny air passages, capillaries and nerve filaments in the bronchi and lungs. This results in all kinds of acute and chronic diseases of the respiratory organs and intensifies oxygen starvation. Here, as in many similar instances, we observe the see-sawing between cause and effect. A disease producing cause sets up a certain ailment. This in turn aggravates and intensifies the primary cause and both together create new troubles, until the entire organism becomes disordered and incapacitated.

Myxoedoma. This ailment is due to more or less complete inactivity of the thyroid gland. The disease is much more frequent in women than in men, mostly in those women who have borne children. The disease is characterized by the accumulation of colloid material in the circulation. This causes capillary obstruction and dropsical swelling. Frequently the hair and eyebrows fall out, the nails and teeth loosen and drop out, while the skin takes on a very peculiar texture and appearance resembling leather. After extirpation, or complete inactivity of the gland through other causes, death follows usually within a week from the manifestation of the first symptom of myxoedema.

Chlorosis, eclampsia, eczema, epilepsy, hysteria and other forms of disease are undoubtedly more or less aggravated by either hyperactivity or inactivity of the thyroid gland. We of the school of Natural Therapeutics have the satisfaction of knowing that even when we do not understand the exact causes and multiform effects and complications of these and other disorders, we can always apply the best treatment possible under the circumstances by overcoming with our natural methods of living and of treatment the three primary manifestations of all physical disease. (See Vol.I, Chap.V.)

Addison's Disease. Synonyms: Melasma, suprarenalis, "the bronzed skin disease" (Fig.32, Area 19, right). Allopathic definition and description: A constitutional disease characterized by degenerative changes in the suprarenal capsules or semilunar ganglia, accompanied by pigmentation of the skin. Causes unknown. There is said to be some connection between Addison's Disease and tuberculosis. Pathological changes are found also in the semilunar ganglia and branches of the sympathetic nerve. The skin assumes a peculiar bronze or blackish pigmentation. The backs of the hands, for instance, look as black as those of a negro, while the inner surface looks pale and white. Duration about two years. Prognosis, incurable. The treatment (as in all cases of chronic disease) must be symptomatic.

Natural Therapeutic Description and Treatment. The adrenals are two little bodies situated one above either kidney. Their function is to supply to the blood certain substances which produce profound effects upon the vital economy of the body. Extirpation or total inactivity of these tiny organs, as well as of the thyroid gland, is followed by rapid decline and death. The secretions of the adrenals have a powerful effect upon all the processes of oxidation in the body. They are to the body what the igniter is to the automobile. As the latter ignites and explodes the gas in the machine, so the secretions of the adrenals in the circulation make possible the combustion of food materials and of morbid waste in the body. The symptoms following the sudden or gradual destruction of the adrenal glands have been named Addison's Disease. The onset is gradual and the patient develops a feeling of weakness and langour. This is followed by extreme muscular prostration. The pulse becomes weak and irregular, with feebleness of the heart's action. Lowered blood pressure is due to the depression of the nerve centres which control the compression of the blood vessels and the heart action. There may be gastro-intestinal disturbances resulting in nausea, vomiting and diarrhoea. The skin becomes bronzed or blackish in appearance. Temperature subnormal.

This ailment is rather rare and occurs mostly in men between twenty and forty years of age. Pressure upon the semilunar ganglia, due to connective tissue adhesions, is a possible cause by creating interferences with the blood supply to the suprarenal bodies. Postmorten examinations have shown that frequently the degeneration of the suprarenal bodies is of a tuberculous nature. When the destructive changes in these ductless glands are too far advanced, even the most thorough natural treatment may fail to arrest the degenerative processes. If, however, the patient is placed under natural treatment during the initial stages of the disease, improvement and cure are sure to follow. We have proved this to be true in many cases. Several patients of this type who came under my observation exhibited drug signs in the iris in the area of the kidneys. The degenerative processes may also be caused or aggravated by interference with the nerve or blood supply through impingement by mechanical lesions or contraction of connective tissues. Thorough systematic natural treatment by all approved methods will meet

and overcome the causes of the disease whatever they may
be, if this is at all possible in the nature of the particular case.
If systemic poisons or poisonous drugs are paralyzing or destroying the glandular structures, natural diet and all methods
which promote elimination of morbid matter and poisons will
bring about the desired improvement. Mechanical lesions and
interference with blood and nerve supply must be corrected
by manipulative treatment. It will be found in such cases that
a diet low in protein and rich in mineral salts is more advisable
than fasting, because the disease itself produces great weakness and emaciation.

Signs of Glandular Lesions in the Iris.
(Fig. 32)

The chronic signs in Fig. 32, right, areas 21 and 15, respectively, showed in the iris of a man of forty-five. He had contracted
several gonorrhoeal infections which had been suppressed in
the usual manner. The sign in 15, right, testes, shows that the
disease and drug poisons caused the atrophy of the sex
glands. This explains why he became impotent within a year
after the disease was "cured". He also suffered since that time
from chronic rheumatism of the arthritic type, especially in
the lower extremities. This is indicated by the chronic signs in
area 18, right and left. In many instances of suppressed
gonorrhoea and syphilis I have noticed that the patients were
sterile (unable to produce offspring) while still capable of performing the sexual act. Many of these cases showed lesions in
area 15, right or left.

The sign of an acute lesion in area 23, right, Fig. 32, was
in a patient who had sustained a severe fall, striking the end of
the spine and bending the coccyx inward. This caused irritation of the coccygeal gland, resulting in inflammation of the
tiny sympathetic ganglion. This in turn caused excruciating
pains, contraction of the sphincter ani, stubborn constipation
and haemorrhoids. Allopathic physicians had recommended
surgical removal of the gland. The coccygeal lesion was
improved by manipulative treatment and the tension relieved
by dilation of the sphincter ani. This overcame the constipation and cured the haemorrhoids.

The chronic lesion in area 23, left. Fig. 32, was visible in the iris of a patient who had suffered for many years with paralysis agitans, the result of mercurial treatment for syphilis early in life. In this case the sphincters of the anus and the bladder were so relaxed that the faeces and urine were discharged involuntarily.

CHAPTER XXIV

BASIC DIAGNOSIS

Introduction.

One of the fundamental principles of the philosophy of Natural Therapeutics is the unity of disease. This means that all the various forms of disease arise from a few primary manifestations, namely, lowered vitality, abnormal composition of vital fluids and accumulation of morbid waste and systemic poisons in the organism. It remains for us to explain why it is possible that in the same kind of an organism a great variety of diseases can arise from a few primary abnormal conditions. To this we answer, it is the organism which is infinitely complex, not the disease. Man, not his disorder, is the great study. Since a few primary causes of disease may produce an infinite multitude of symptoms, it is impossible accurately to diagnose the underlying disease from external symptoms. Therefore, basic diagnosis does not attempt the diagnosis of symptoms, but aims at the diagnosis of the patient. When we understand the organism, the functions and interdependence of its parts and organs, disease offers but a simple problem. All men are not alike. All men do not function alike. They are alike only in general anatomical structure — only in crude form or mould. Man is not altogether a machine operating on mechanical principles. Closely allied with the mechanical structure, and controlling it, are the vital or psychical and the mental or intellectual principles.

The numerous functions of the human body may conveniently be classified under three main groups, namely, respiration, alimentation and generation.

Respiration is that function which takes care of the oxygenation of the blood and the elimination of burned carbonaceous materials through the lungs. As explained in Vol.II of this series, in the chapter dealing with correct breathing, respiration is the function on which depends the inflow of the dynamic force or life force necessary to maintain the vital activities within the body.

Alimentation is that function which enables the body to digest and assimilate the proper quantity and quality of food, and which removes the residue of such processes from the body.

Generation is that function which assures perpetuity to the human race by means of reproduction. The secretions of the ductless glands of the generative organs are necessary to the maintenace of the vital activities of the organism.

Back of these three basic functions of the human organism lie three corresponding life principles — the physical material principle, the mental or intellectual principle and the psychical or moral principle. The material principle stands for substance, solidity, physique, and is closely allied to the terrestrial plane. This principle is in sympathy with physical nature, and its nerve mechanism — the great sympathetic — is the instrument through which the life force controls animal functions. The one who possesses a large proportion of this principle is hardier, stronger and more robust than those in whom either the mental or psychical principle predominates. The psychical or moral principle connects us with the psyche or soul of the universe. Through the psychic principle the individual consciousness receives an influx of intuitive intelligence and creative will from the great creative Intelligence which some call God or Nature, others Cosmic Intelligence, Creative Will, Over-Soul, Brahm, and by many other names. The psychic "wireless" is therefore the source of inspiration and illumination; it makes possible the apprehension of abstract truth, — of time and space, of right and wrong. It is the "light that lighteth every man that cometh into the world".

Consciousness is the passive capacity of the individual intelligence, soul or ego. It receives impressions and impulses.

from two sources — from the physical material surroundings through the sensory organs, and from the immaterial psychical world of laws and causes through the psychic principle. Through the psychic wireless it receives an influx of intuitive intelligence and creative will. This innate intelligence senses, observes and compares the sensory impressions and sensations, and discriminates between them. It classifies the contents of consciousness and from them draws conclusions and judgements. Thus originates and grows the reasoning mind. From this it will be seen that the mind is that principle which stands between and connects the physical and psychical principles, and that we create it ourselves. The mind has been likened to a circle, the centre of which is the ego and the circumference of which may be anywhere in the universe. In the new born infant or in the idiot the diameter is exceedingly limited, while in the great scientist or philisopher it may fathom the secrets of the starry heavens. It does not reach full completion until it embraces all there is to be known in the sidereal universe. Its expansion depends upon the number and variety of sensory impressions and impulses received from the physical or spiritual (material) surroundings and upon the amount of thinking, reasoning and philosophizing brought to bear upon the contents of consciousness. These psychological phonographic and photographic films constitue memory and the subconscious mind of the psychologists and occultists. Sensory impressions and impulses from without and the thinking and reasoning from within, give rise to sensations, emotions, impulses and desires which, in turn call forth the activity of the will. The will in action is volition.

What nerve specialists and psychologists call the reflex arc consists of this twofold function of receiving and giving, which underlies all the activities of human life. The balancing of receiving and giving constitute physical health as well as intellectual, moral and social health. Violations of nature's laws in all domains of life and action involve the violation of this basic principle of giving and receiving which is the law of compensation in operation. On it depends the preservation of energy; it is the basis of civil as well as of ethical and moral law. Only by complying with its demands can we solve the

social problem. Reason and common sense should tell us that
the relationships of human life must be under the control of
natural law as well as the relationships of numbers, of atoms
of matter and the harmonics of sound. This is true notwithstanding the assertion of materialistic philosophy that
there is nothing innately settled and permanent about ethics
and morals, that they are subject to change and custom like
fashions in hats, frocks and walking canes.

From the foregoing it becomes apparent that the mental
or intellectual principle comprises the faculties which constitute the reasoning or objective mind, such as observation,
discrimination, calculation, deduction and logic. It harbours
the executive qualities and prompts voluntary action. It is a
thinking apparatus and, in itself, is cold, calculating and
exact. It is the seat of judgement apart from sentiment and
feeling, and moderates the qualities of sympathy and mercy.
The reasoning or objective mind deals only with facts and
data gathered from observation and experience. This is in
agreement with materialistic and monistic science and
philosophy; but these systems leave out of consideration that
which makes thinking, reasoning and philosophizing a
possibility, namely, the psychic principle. While studying
and explaining the phenomena of life, they try to exclude life
itself from the scheme of things.

In the limited space of this treatise I can deal only very
briefly with the relationships between the intellectual and
psychic principles and the brain and nervous system. I have
elaborated this in detail in Vol.IV of this series, dealing with
natural eugenics. Here we shall trace briefly the relationship
of the three basic principles to the physical organism. The
three basic principles of the human entity herein described
sustain a definite relationship to the three principle divisions
of the great brain or cerebrum, and through these to the three
basic functions of the organism already described. It should
be understood that these correspondences or relationships
have nothing to do with the location of phrenological centres.
Long continued careful observation and practical experience
have revealed the fact that the three main divisions of the
cerebrum and the three basic functions of alimentation, respiration and generation are closely allied and interdependent.

The Great Brain.

By Dr. W.F. Havard

The cerebrum is divided into two hemispheres, occupying the greater part of the cranial cavity which is formed by the union of the bones of the skull. Each hemisphere is divided by deep fissures into three separate portions called lobes. They are named according to their location in reference to the bones of the skull which form their outer protection, as follows: the occipito-temporal lobes, the parietal lobes and the frontal lobes. The occipito-temporal lobes are the seat of the material or the physical principle; the parietal lobes are the seat of the psychical or moral principle, and the frontal lobes are the seat of the mental or intellectual functions. The following illustration will serve to show these different areas of the brain.

The degree of development in the various brain areas will determind the relative strenght of the three basic principle in any one individual. For instance, a person possessing the greatest brain development in the occipito-temporal lobes of the brain is of the physical type, while a person with a high, straight, prominent forehead with the greatest brain development in the frontal lobes, is placed in the intellectual class. The person who has his greatest and best development in the parietal region, or at the topmost portion of the head belongs to the moral class. The classification of individuals in this manner makes it possible to determine the relative strength of the various organ systems. The main organ systems, as we

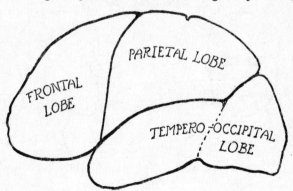

Fig. 1. Side view of cerebrum, showing lobes and fissures.

PHYSICAL BASE

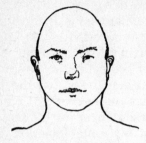 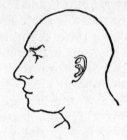

Full Temples   Well developed
                       occipital lobes

MORAL BASE

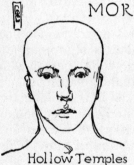 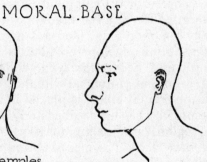

Hollow Temples   High top head

MENTAL BASE

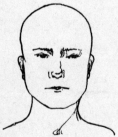 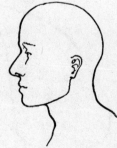

High square forehead   Straight forehead

Fig. 2.

have seen, are the digestive, respiratory and generative, and
there is a direct correspondence between the brain development and the strength of the three basic physiological functions. Good development in the physical brain region
(occipito-temporal lobes) establishes the fact that the individual possesses strong digestive action. The development of the
moral portion of the brain (parietal lobes) determines the
strength of generative action, while the degree of development in the mental portion of the brain (frontal lobes) will
determine the strength of the respiratory action. The ideal
human being, of course, would be one in whom these three
principles were balanced; or in other words, in whom the
mental, moral and physical portions of the brain were equally
developed. Such individuals, however, are of rare occurrence. The more nearly equal these three principles are in
development and vitality in any one individual the more perfect he is — mentally, morally and physically.

No person today could be totally lacking in any one of
these principles without being marked as a defective. If the
physical principle is very weak he will not survive infancy. If
the intellect, or the frontal lobes, are only slightly developed
he will be an idiot. If the psychical or moral area is
undeveloped the person lacks intuition and imagination, and
is therefore limited in inventive and creative ability. Such a
person is lacking in the intuitive perception of moral, ethical
and religious principles. If, on the other hand, the psychical
principle greatly predominates over the intellectual the person tends to emotionalism, is negative and subjective to outside influences and becomes an easy prey to hypnotic and
mediumistic control. Everyone must possess the three basic
qualities to some degree, and the proportion of them determines not only a person's habits and characteristics, his likes
and dislikes, and his general temperament, but also his sus-
ceptibility to abnormalities and diseases of one form or
another. That portion of the brain which shows the greatest
development in any one individual is called the "base", while
the two weaker areas are called the "inclinations", the
stronger being the "first" and the weaker the "second" inclination. The greater the development of the inclinations the more
difficult it becomes to determine the base. The base is there,

however, and is the foundation on which the person is built.
The base has a definite value, and the inclinations are relative
to it. The latter may both be very weak or they may both be
strong, or one may be strong and the other weak. All degrees
of development occur; no two individuals are exactly alike.
Where both inclinations are of a low degree of development,
the base is more pronounced by contrast.

As we have shown, each principle has its particular correlated group of organs and functions in the body. These are
known as the fundamental organs, and the organ which corresponds to a person's basic principle becomes his basic
organ. For example, if someone is physically based, his basic
organ is the liver, which is the principal organ of the digestive
system. The liver of that person is the strongest organ in his
body, and is the one on which he depends to the largest degree
for his support. In a morally based individual the generative
organs are the strongest; while in a mentally based person the
lungs are the organ upon which that person depends for his
main support. There is no limit to the combinations that can
be made with these three principles, any more than there is a
limit to the number of shades which can be derived through
the mixture of the three basic colours, red, blue and yellow.
By determining as nearly as possible the base of a person and
the relative strength of his inclinations, we are able to gauge
his individual index.

By individual index we mean the relative degree of
activity on the part of the three principle organ systems under
normal conditions. So, for example, a person who is
materially based with a first moral inclination and a second
intellectual inclination, is strongest in the digestive organs.
His greatest weakness lies in the lungs, while the generative
organs are intermediate. From this it follows that disease processes will manifest first in the weakest organ or groups of
organs which belong to the second inclination. Next to succumb will be the organs of first inclination. The chances for
recovery are good as long as the basic organ and its aids are in
fair condition and able to compensate for the weakness and
deficiencies of the organs of the first and second inclinations.
When, however, the organism becomes weakened and diseased at its base or foundation, then the superstructure will

soon give way and succumb to nature's destructive processes. Thus basic diagnosis aids the physician to locate the organs of least resistance and thereby the seat of the disease, as well as to estimate the chances of recovery. For instance, as long as a person with a strong physical base is endowed with good digestive power and assimilation, disorders of the respiratory and generative organs will be easily overcome, but when the liver, stomach and intestines of such a person become seriously affected by degenerative processes, then destruction in the lungs or kidneys will soon result in fatal termination. Thus basic diagnosis enables the physician to express a more accurate opinion as to whether the case will improve, or whether there will be a continued decline. It also enables him to determine which organ system needs the greatest attention from a therapeutic standpoint.

Application of Basic Diagnosis.
Correspondences Between Brain Areas and Organic Functions.

Occipito-temporal lobes (lower portion of cerebrum) — Digestive System

Parietal lobes (top portion of cerebrum) — Generative System

Frontal lobes (front portion of cerebrum) — Respiratory System

It is only in rare cases and in exceptionally well developed individuals that we find all three brain regions and consequently all three organ systems developed to an equal degree and capable of exercising the same degree of function. In the vast majority of people at least one of these organs systems is markedly weaker than the other two. When disease begins to affect anyone it is this weaker group of organs which first begins to manifest changes in function and ultimately in structure. To describe all the changes as they occur and the manner in which a disease process progresses, and how and why it is reflected from one part of the organism to another, would require the writing of a special volume on this subject alone. To prove these facts would necessitate the recitation of the life histories of a long list of cases from which these statements have been verified. Enough has been given to enable the physician and the intelligent layman to continue the study of this interesting subject and to profit by its practical application.

To recapitulate: As a disease process develops, the resistance of the weaker organs is broken down first and the condition is then carried to the next stronger group of organs, and finally to the strongest or basic organ. When the disease process reaches the basic organ, the patient has entered upon the last stages of pathological change. If the disease process continues unchecked he will finally succumb as disease destroys his stronghold.

In the following illustrations only the general types of people will be considered. There are six general types classified according to their bases and inclinations. The base represents the strongest system; the first inclination, the system of intermediate strength; the second inclination, the weakest organ system.

1. General Physical Type. (Fig.3)

(A) Base, physical; first inclination, moral; second inclination, mental.

In this case the strongest organs are the digestive; the basic organ the liver. The intermediate organs are the reproductive (generative glands and the system of ductless glands); the weakest organs are the lungs. Prominent symptoms and preliminary healing crises are those emanating from the generative organs and the ductless glands

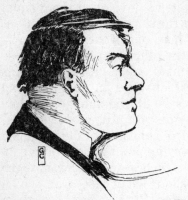 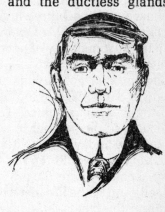

Fig. 3.

(thyroid, suprarenals, pituitary) in cases where the disease changes have not yet reached the basic organ. Diseases likely to prove fatal if not checked in time, or if improperly treated, are those producing destructive changes in the digestive organs, and in the liver — diabetes, cancer of the liver, cirrhosis of the liver, and advanced Bright's disease. Early symptoms of failure of the liver manifest themselves in the form of rheumatism, which may be reflected to the heart. Prognosis is good in cases where destructive changes have not yet occurred in the liver. In other words, where the principle symptoms are in the intermediate organs and the liver is still capable of compensating for the functional failure of other organs, this patient still has a chance to retrace his steps and recover his health under natural treatment. In this case the liver, in its endeavour to compensate, may increase its activity to such a degree that symptoms will arise. These symptoms, however, are functional and should not be considered alarming. It is only when the liver's function begins to fail, due to destructive changes in that organ, that the prognosis becomes rather grave. The treatment should be general natural therapeutic treatment and such natural methods as can be directed especially to the liver for the purpose of relieving it of work or of increasing its functional activity, the first purpose being to maintain compensation in the basic organ. The most vitally essential part of such treatment consists of periods of rational fasting, interspersed with periods of strict

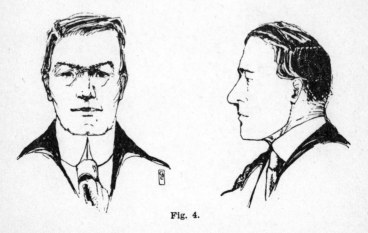

Fig. 4.

eliminative diet until the liver has had the opportunity to cleanse the blood stream of surplus waste products.

(B) (Fig.4) Base, physical; first inclination, mental; second inclination, moral.

In this case the strongest organs are the digestive; the basic organ the liver. The intermediate organs are the lungs; the weakest organs are the reproductive and the system of ductless glands. Prominent symptoms and healing crises are those emanating from the respiratory organs, in cases where the disease changes have not yet reached the liver. The diseases likely to prove fatal, the prognosis and the treatment indicated are the same as in Type A.

2. General Moral Type.

(A) (Fig.5) Base, moral; first inclination, physical; second inclination, mental.

In this case the strongest organs are the ductless glands; the basic organs generative or reproductive. The intermediate organs are the digestive and the weakest organs the lungs. Prominent symptoms and preliminary healing crises are those emanating from the digestive organs and liver. Diseases likely to prove fatal are those producing destructive changes in the generative organs which result in degenerative changes in the system. The prognosis is good unless destructive changes have taken place in the generative glands. In persons of the moral type, functional symptoms manifest themselves in the nervous system as a result of increased activity in the

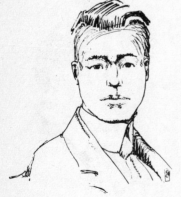
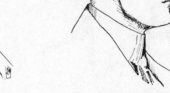

Fig. 5.

ductless glands. This is largely due to the endeavour of these structures to compensate for deficiencies in the intermediate and weakest organs. It is when this compensatory action begins to fail and destructive changes are noticeable in the nervous system that the outlook becomes grave. The treatment should be general natural treatment directed particularly to the generative organs for the purpose of maintaining compensation. A strict eliminative diet must be adhered to and occasional fasts of from three to seven days duration. Sun baths should be employed with the sun's rays directed to the pelvic region. The remainder of the body should be protected during this specific treatment. Such a sun bath should not be prolonged above fifteen minutes. The vital fluids of patients of this type must be conserved, consequently there must be total abstinence from sexual intercourse during the period of their cure.

(B) (Fig.6) Base, moral; first inclination, mental; second inclination, physical.

In this case the strongest organs are the ductless glands; basic organs, generative. The intermediate organs are the respiratory and the weakest the digestive. Prominent symptoms and preliminary healing crises are those emanating from the respiratory organs, in cases where the disease changes have not yet reached the ductless glands and the nervous system. Diseases likely to prove fatal, prognosis and treatment are the same as for Type 2 A.

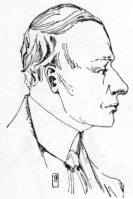 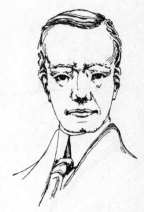

Fig. 6.

3. General Mental Type.

(A) (Fig.7) Base, mental; first inclination, physical; second inclination, moral.

In this case the strongest are the lungs; basic organ upper lobes. The intermediate organs are the digestive and the weakest the ductless glands. Prominent symptoms and preliminary healing crises are those emanating from the digestive organs, in cases where destructive changes have not yet occurred in the lungs. Diseases likely to prove fatal if improperly treated are those producing destructive changes in the lungs, the chief of which is tuberculosis. The prognosis is good in cases where destructive changes have not occurred in the lungs. The treatment should be general natural treatment with a strict eliminative diet and frequent fasts of short duration. Outdoor exercises are necessary for people of this type, particularly such as will increase the respiratory action and maintain sufficient compensation through the lungs, so as to enable the intermediate and weakest organs to recover their tone and return to a higher state of function.

(B) (Fig.8) Base, mental; first inclination, moral; second inclination, physical.

In this case the strongest organs are the lungs; basic organ, upper lobes. The intermediate organs are the ductless glands, the weakest the digestive organs. Prominent symptoms and preliminary healing crises are those emanating from the ductless glands and nervous system, in cases where des-

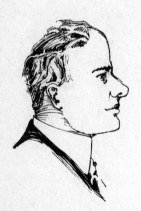
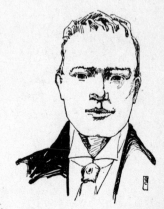

Fig. 7.

tructive changes have not yet occurred in the lungs. Diseases likely to prove fatal, prognosis and treatment are the same as for Type 3 A.

From the foregoing outline it will be seen that the prominent symptoms occur in the organs of the first inclination. This needs a slight explanation. During the growing and developing years of a person — the years before eighteen — symptomatic conditions are likely to arise from the organs of the second inclination, the severity depending upon the strength of these organs or their degree of resistance. Crisis conditions frequently manifest themselves through these organs during this period of life. If they are very weak, however, and the person is living under unfavourable or unhygienic conditions, symptoms will begin to appear in the organs of the first inclination about the age of puberty. It is through the organs of the first or stronger inclination that we must expect a crisis to occur during the process of cure; for the production of a crisis not only requires resistive power in the part selected for this activity, but also that some other part shall maintain sufficient strength to carry on the necessary compensation. Where the crisis occurs through the organs of the stronger inclination, the basic organ carries the compensation. If the disease process actually reaches the basic organ, having already progressed through the weakest and intermediate organs, a crisis cannot take place in the basic organ, because there is nothing left to take up the compensatory activities.

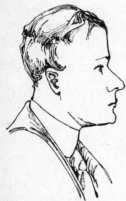 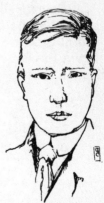

Fig. 8.

In order to arrive at a correct basic diagnosis we must first of all determine in which of the three brain areas the greatest development lies. It becomes necessary then for us to make a general study of heads. If from the front view of a person we gather the information that both temples are well developed and full, and the line of the head from the angle of the orbit over the ears and around the occiput or base of the brain shows the greatest development of any part of the head, we place that person in the physical class. His base determined, the inclinations then receive our attention. The higher and straighter the forehead, the more development exists in the frontal lobes of the brain, the more mentality is possessed by that person. If the forehead, then, contains greater development than the topmost portion of the head (parietal region), then the person's first inclincation is mental, and his second moral. If, on the other hand, the parietal region contains a more marked development, is larger and better proportioned, then the person's first inclination is moral, and his second mental. Let us take another example: Looking at a person from the front, his temples appear to be hollow, and the line round the base of the head appears to be constricted. Immediately we know that he cannot be physically based; he must then be either morally or mentally based. We now take a profile view and we find that the forehead recedes slightly, consequently he cannot be mentally based. The parietal region, however, is well developed and therefore he belongs to the moral type. Coming back to the front view, we find a high, well developed forehead, which impresses us as having a greater value than the development existing over the temples and at the base of the brain; so we pronounce his first inclination to be mental, and his second inclination is then physical.

CHAPTER 1
IRIDOLOGY
pp 15-23

This chapter draws attention to the uncertainty and incompleteness of the methods of diagnosis usually employed and points out the importance of iridiagnosis and Spinal Analysis in enabling diagnosis and prognosis to be greatly improved. The history of iridiagnosis is traced from its first discovery by Von Peokzely in the second half of the 10th century and its development by a number of pioneers in Europe and America. The nervous and circulatory mechanism by which signs in the iris are produced is discussed.

CHAPTER II
ANATOMY OF THE IRIS
pp 25-29

The anatomy, history and physiology of the iris is discussed with a number of anatomical illustrations. It is explained that the normal colour of the iris is either light blue or light brown and the reason for this is given.

CHAPTER III
EXPLANATION OF THE KEY TO IRIDOLOGY
pp 31-33

This chapter is an explanation of the chart forming the frontispiece of the volume and this is based on the discovery of the areas in the iris which correspond with the various organs and parts of the body. Marks and discolourations in parts of the iris are evidences of changes having taken place in the corresponding organs or parts of the body or to the deposit in those parts of substances which are foreign to the body or uncongenial to it.

CHAPTER IV

A UNIFORM DIVISION AND CLASSIFICATION OF DISEASE
pp 39-45

For the facilitation of the diagnosis and treatment of chronic disease it is possible to distinguish four distinct 'stages of encumbrance', each with their distinctive signs in the iris. These are (1) the hereditary congenital stage, (2) the acute and subacute inflammatory stage, (3) the chronic stage and (4) the chronic destructive stage. The prognosis in a given case will very much depend on the 'stage of encumbrance' present and the importance of the organs involved.

CHAPTER V

DENSITY OF THE IRIS
pp 47-58

Definition and cause of Density. Illustration (Fig.6) showing four degrees of density corresponding to the 'stages of encumbrance'. Density is a guide to stamina, vital resistance to disease, recuperative power and expectancy of life. Closed lesions, lymphatic rosary, arsenic signs and radii solaris are discussed.

CHAPTER VI

NERVE RINGS
pp 59-66

These and the 'sympathetic wreath' are concentric white rings present in varying degrees which are indicative of acute nervous activity (Figs.7 and 7a) and also give evidence of the iris being divided into zones. During treatment such white signs appearing in the iris often indicate the approach of a healing crisis. In cases of constipation the state of the sympathetic wreath assists in diagnosis as to whether the constipation is spastic or flacid, thus influencing the type of treatment which is appropriate. See case report and Fig.8 on pp.65 and 68.

CHAPTER VII

THE SCURF RIM
pp 67-73

The presence of the dark 'Scurf Rim' often seen round the outside border of the iris is the sign of the skin being in a weak, enervated, atonic or anaemic and atrophic condition and so being unable to fulfil its proper functions as an eliminative organ and as part of the temperature response and regulation mechanism. The principal causes of this, are suppression of all kinds of skin eruptions from childhood onwards and the coddling of the skin by a failure to expose it to the stimulation of air, sunlight and cold water.

CHAPTER VIII

ITCH OR PSORA SPOTS IN THE IRIS
pp 75-88

The brown itch or psora spots which appear in many eyes are also due to the suppression of eczema, skin eruptions and parasitic infestations (scabies, etc.) and are of more serious import than the scurf rim alone. The term 'psora' which was used by Hahnemann, the founder of homeopathy, to cover the 'scrofulous diathesis' resulting largely from suppression of skin conditions, often over many generations, which was regarded by him as being the basis of many chronic diseases as, for instance, leprosy and cancer. Lindlahr here gives a number of quotations from Hahnemann's writings setting forth his theory of psora and his opposition to the suppressive treatment of skin conditions. He also gives interesting case reports.

CHAPTER IX

COMPARISON OF FERMENTATION TO INFLAMMATION
pp 89-106

Lindlahr here draws a comparison between fermentation and inflammation, both being processes of oxidation or combustion accompanied by increased chemical activity and temperature. These processes are normally self-limiting and essentially beneficial but if interfered with the results can be serious. Acute inflammatory reactions in the body if rightly guided lead to improvement and cure but if suppressed lead to chronic disease. An illustrative case report is given.

CHAPTER X
SIGNS OF INORGANIC MINERALS IN THE IRIS OF THE EYE
pp 108-122

Lindlahr here shows that substances congenial to the body and normally belonging to it do not produce signs and discolourations in the iris, whereas foreign substances do. Even chemical elements which are congenial or necessary to the body economy will produce signs and will cause damage if taken in inorganic form. There are two full page plates attached to this chapter. One of these gives the signs to be found in the iris in the different stages of encumbrance (see Chapter V); the other, which is in colour, gives examples of eyes which are very much discoloured owing to drug poisonings of various kinds. There are special discussions of the signs of iron, sodium, potassium, calcium and magnesium in inorganic form. The allopathic uses of iron in various combinations and its toxicology are discussed.

CHAPTER XI
SIGNS OF POISONS IN THE EYE
pp 123-129

Poison signs in the eyes showing the presence of such alteratives as mercury, iodine and arsenic are sometimes difficult to explain. This may be because the patient does not remember ever having taken remedies containing such substances, but also many poisons are absorbed as the result of industrial processes or the adulteration of foods with colouring matter or preservatives.

CHAPTER XII

MERCURY, HYDRARGYRUM OR QUICKSILVER
pp 131-147

This chapter gives information on the allopathic uses of mercurial preparations in Lindlahr's time, especially in the treatment of syphilis, and on common sources of accidental mercurial poisoning. The toxicology and symptoms of mercurial poisoning are given as well as the signs in the iris and the common ways in which the drug can be eliminated in 'healing crises' during treatment. The use of mercurial preparations in the treatment of syphilis which was then almost universal is discussed at length and many quotations are given from the writings of Dr. Hermann who was the specialist in the great hospital for the treatment of venereal diseases in Vienna. Dr. Lindlahr followed Dr. Hermann in regarding syphilis as an ordinary acute disease and in treating it with success by simple natural methods. Tertiary syphilis was regarded by both of them as the result of treatment by mercury or other alteratives.

CHAPTER XIII

CINCHONA — QUININE
pp 149-159

The signs in the iris, allopathic uses, accidental poisonings, and toxicology of quinine are given and the forms of elimination to be expected in 'healing crises' are noted. The use of quinine in the prevention and treatment of malaria (and other conditions) is discussed and evidence is given, with case reports, of how malaria can be prevented and cured without the use of quinine.

CHAPTER XIV

IODINE
pp 161-168

The signs in the iris, allopathic uses, accidental poisonings and toxicology of iodine are discussed and the forms of elimination to be expected in 'healing crises' are noted. Lindlahr discusses the description of iodine in medical and homoeopathic texts and gives case reports including his own personal experience. Common symptoms of iodism are given.

CHAPTER XV
LEAD
pp 169-171

The signs in the iris, allopathic uses, accidental poisonings and toxicology of lead are discussed, common symptoms of plumbism are given, and forms of elimination to be expected in 'healing crises' are noted. Several case reports are given.

CHAPTER XVI
ARSENIC
pp 173-177

Signs in the iris, allopathic uses, accidental poisonings and toxicology of arsenic are given and discussed. Common symptoms of chronic arsenic poisoning and the forms of elimination to be expected in 'healing crises' are noted. Case reports are given.

CHAPTER XVII
BROMIDES
pp 179-187

Signs in the iris, allopathic uses and toxicology of bromides are given. Common symptoms of bromism and the forms of elimination to be expected in 'healing crises' are noted. The special affinity of bromides for brain and nervous tissue is noted. The discovery of the 'epilectic centre' in the cerebellum and the possibility of influencing this by surgery in some cases are discussed, but the harmfulness of the treatment of epilepsy by bromides and their use as sedatives, hypnotics, antispasmodics, etc., in various mental and nervous conditions are condemned. A number of case reports are given.

CHAPTER XVIII
COAL TAR PRODUCTS
pp 189-192

Lindlahr discusses the use of acetanilid, antipyrine, creosote, phenaticin, antikamnia and other coal tar derivatives as pain killers, hypnotics, antipyretics, or 'germ killers'. He mentions also the common use of coal tar products in the colouring and preserving of certain foods. The signs in the iris, allopathic uses, toxicology and common symptoms of coal tar poisoning are given. The forms of elimination to be expected in 'healing crises' are noted.

CHAPTER XIX
MISCELLANEOUS DRUGS
pp 193-202

This chapter gives information about salicylic acid, strychnine, phosphorus, turpentine, glycerine, ergot, opiates and narcotics, opium, laudanum, paregoric, morphine, cocaine, anodynes and analgesics, sedatives and hypnotics. The general plan is that the signs in the iris, allopathic uses, the symptoms of poisoning, toxicology and the forms of elimination to be expected in 'healing crises' are given for each drug. Finally Lindlahr makes a plea for the non-use of opiates even in cases of terminal illnesses which are usually accompanied with great suffering and declares that under natural care the suffering is less and the end more peaceful.

CHAPTER XX
DISEASES OF THE VITAL ORGANS — THEIR SIGNS IN THE IRIS
pp 203-218

This chapter deals very fully with diseases of the most important vital organs — stomach and intestines, liver and spleen, kidneys and lungs. Numerous illustrations are given of the irides of persons suffering from various degrees of pathological change in these organs and the case histories which accompany the illustrations trace how the deteriorated conditions have arisen from the accumulation of pathological encumbrances in the body and suppression, mostly by drugs, of the attempts of the organism to improve its health and performance. Lindlahr's explanation of the function of the spleen and his rejection of the general acceptance of the idea of phagocytosis as put forward by Metchnikoff and also his contention that micro-organisms should be regarded as the accompaniments or results of disease rather than its cause are of great interest and importance.

CHAPTER XXI
CHRONIC DISEASES — THEIR SIGNS IN THE IRIS
pp 219-231

This chapter deals with a number of chronic diseases such as asthma, psora, diabetes, Bright's disease and diseases of the sexual organs. A number of case reports and the findings in the iris in such cases are given.

CHAPTER XXII
THE DUCTLESS GLANDS AND THEIR SECRETIONS
pp 233-241

This chapter gives an account of the ductless glands and discusses their functions and their interrelationships. There are extensive quotations from the works of Dr. Charles E. de Sejous who was a well known authority on the subject in Lindlahr's time. It may be said that Lindlahr's account may be in certain respects out of date but he agrees with Sejous as to the importance of the endocrine system and particularly of the pituitary, adrenal and thyroid glands. On the proper functioning of the endocrine system the growth and development of the body and mind and the power of the body to cope with toxicity and disease are largely based and controlled. When it comes to treatment Lindlahr does not believe in the use of drugs or of hormonal extracts derived from animals except perhaps as a temporary expedient in certain cases. He contends that the best results can be got by all round natural treatment including specific manipulation to improve blood and nerve supply to the organs concerned. See also chapter XXIII.

CHAPTER XXIII
DISEASES OF THE DUCTLESS GLANDS — THEIR SIGNS IN THE IRIS
pp 243-255

Hyper-thyroidism or Goitre, of the soft, hard and exophthalmic types, are discussed, also thyroid deficiency, myxoedema and

Addison's Disease. The natural and allopathic treatment of these conditions is compared and contrasted. Lindlahr is firmly opposed to any form of drug treatment, to the use of hormonal extracts derived from animals which, he says, causes the gland to deteriorate further and more rapidly and to surgery of the thyroid. He maintains that all round natural treatment will have better results than the allopathic treatments generally used and will produce a complete cure in many cases if taken in time. While the removal of 'foci of infection' may be an important factor in some endocrine troubles these should not be dealt with by surgery but by natural treatment. There are illustrations of signs in the iris and case reports of some cases are given.

CHAPTER XXIV

BASIC DIAGNOSIS
pp 257-272

Basic Diagnosis is a form of diagnosis not now much used but it was believed in by Dr. Lindlahr and was used by him in combination with Iridiagnosis. The technique is based on the belief and discovery that all human beings are of one of three basic types, that is that they are physically, psychically or mentally based. Which is a person's basic type can be diagnosed by the relative size and development of the temporo-occipital, parietal and frontal lobes of the cranium. Persons of each type have certain organs which are naturally basic and strong and others which are comparatively weak and vulnerable. In treating a chronic condition whether the patients's basic organs are affected or not may have an important bearing on the prognosis. In short, the type of body which a patient has may need to be considered as well as the pathological findings.